Early Praise for

From Hoarding to Hope:
Understanding People Who Hoard and How to Help Them

"This is the book I've been waiting for. *From Hoarding to Hope* offers a straightforward, compassionate and practical guide for people who live or work with hoarding disorder."

– Susan Stone, MSW, LCSW, MBA
President, New England Chapter, National Association of Professional Organizers

"I could not put this book down. It's a must read for all human services employees who will be exposed to hoarding disorder."

– Pamela Woodbury
Director, Spencer, MA Council on Aging

"*From Hoarding to Hope* helps clinicians and coaches 'get' the disorder and understand where it has its greatest functional impact. It's a must-have for clinicians' and coaches' reference libraries."

– David D. Nowell, PhD
Clinical Neuropsychologist

"I recommend this book to anyone interested in learning more about hoarding disorder, whether it's for yourself, a friend or in your role as a professional organizer, mental health professional or social worker."

– Rachel Seavey
Professional Organizer

"Geralin Thomas does a great job navigating client stories with firsthand knowledge to provide brutally honest insights that can help anyone who needs to know where to start."

– Matt Paxton
Author & Extreme Cleaner

"*From Hoarding to Hope* is destined to become a staple for a very wide audience. It's an instant classic."

– Standolyn Robertson CPO-CD
Past President, National Association of Professional Organizers (NAPO)

"Ms. Thomas's consultation with various experts around the area of hoarding provides an excellent exploration of the hoarding disorder itself. This will be an important guide for caregivers."

– Rev. Dr. Bonnie L. Prizio, DMIN, LMHC, CLSC
Director, New Hope Counseling Center

"A comprehensive guide to helping people with hoarding disorder. Geralin Thomas's inside perspective on working in hoarding situations is invaluable."

– Janine Adams, CPO, CPO-CD
Past President, St. Louis Chapter, National Association of Professional Organizers

"Bringing together stories from people whose lives have been hijacked by hoarding, Geralin shares her focused insight as well as contributions from other professionals in the field. I highly recommend this book."

Mark Pfeffer LMFT
Director, The Panic Anxiety Recovery Center (PARC)

"Geralin Thomas's book provides the insight needed by many in the caregiving and social services sectors as they encounter hoarding in clients' homes."

– Kimberly Marie Harmon, BSN, RN
Author & Healthcare Consultant

"A must-read for friends, family or even professionals who truly want to help a loved one or client struggling with hoarding disorder."

– Kara Russelo Cline
Professional Organizer

"*From Hoarding to Hope* offers an easy-to-read, compassionate, and thoughtful approach to helping those struggling with clutter and hoarding."

– Robin Zasio, PsyD, LCSW
Director, The Compulsive Hoarding Center

From Hoarding to Hope: Understanding People Who Hoard and How to Help Them

edited by Geralin Thomas

MetroZing Publishing
From Hoarding to Hope: Understanding People Who Hoard and How to Help Them
Edited by Geralin Thomas

Copyright © 2015 by Geralin Thomas
All Rights Reserved

All rights reserved. No part of this publication may be reproduced, distributed, or transmitted in any form or by any means, including photocopying, recording, or other electronic or mechanical methods, without the prior written permission of the publisher, except in the case of brief quotations embodied in critical reviews and certain other noncommercial uses permitted by copyright law. For permission requests, write to the publisher, addressed "Attention: Permissions Coordinator," at the address below.

>MetroZing Publishing
>92 Cornerstone Drive
>Cary, NC 27519

ISBN   978-1506148359
        1506148352

Library of Congress Control Number: 2015905313
CreateSpace, Independent Publishing Platform, North Charleston, SC

*For my husband, Bill,
and my sons, Cole and Chris*

Acknowledgements

This book would not have been possible without the help of many who have generously shared their time, knowledge, and experience with me.

In particular, I thank my organizing colleague *Susan Terkanian* for her unwavering support regarding every aspect of this book—administrative assistant, connector, collaborator, detail maven, researcher extraordinaire, and accountability partner.

The therapists who've contributed to this book and my blog: By generously sharing knowledge and answering my calls, emails, and curious questions, you've helped me and my clients tremendously. You have a gift for taking exceedingly complicated topics and clarifying them brilliantly.

Screaming Flea Productions: Being part of the crew has been very special; thank you for the many opportunities to work with a variety of clients in locations around the country. And, special thanks to the brave people who opened their homes and lives while filming *Hoarders*. You've earned respect and compassion, and best of all, there are many who benefit from your courage.

Assistants, Researchers, Friends, and Organizers: Shawndra Holmberg, Donna Smallin Kuper, Julie Bestry, and Janine Adams: You have gone above and beyond the call of duty when it comes to helping; sharing insider secrets about the deep, dark, mysterious world of writing, editing, and publishing. Thank you for being so generous and willing to spill the beans. I'm grateful for your wisdom.

Standolyn Robertson, Jeri Redman, Kara Cline, and Margaret Lukens: Thanks for being my readers and sounding boards. Your tender compassion with clients is commendable and sets an example for others. Your opinions mean a lot to me. I appreciate your dependability and honest, constructive feedback. *Helena Alkhas, Ellen Delap, and Julie Corracio*: Thanks for keeping it real while simultaneously being optimistic cheerleaders with sunny dispositions.

The NAPO and ICD colleagues I met while assembling teams of volunteers for *Hoarders* shoots: Wow—you worked hard, long days with no complaints and no judgment. You toiled in extreme temperatures, and more often than not, in unpleasant and uncomfortable situations and circumstances. Your dedication and camaraderie amaze me.

My family: I would especially like to thank my husband, Bill Thomas, and my two handsome, intelligent, and charming sons, Cole and Chris (remember, I'm a mom and can brag if I want to). I'm grateful for your encouragement and understanding, but most of all I appreciate you for giving me time away from home to travel, work, and research. Spending nights and weekends away wasn't easy, but your constant encouragement enabled me to learn a lot and be part of something unique.

And, last but not least, I acknowledge those who've helped me write this book and learn more about this disorder than I imagined possible: the clients I've worked with who cope with mild to severe hoarding disorder and hoarding tendencies. Your personal stories, your homes, your courage and curiosity, your vulnerability, and your trust in me have made me a better person and a better organizer. Without you, this book wouldn't be possible. I've learned to respect and appreciate the journeys you've traveled. By sharing your stories, you will help people who want to be helped. Your stories help others understand that there is hope. Thank you!

Contents

Foreword i
Introduction iii

Part 1. The Face of Hoarding Disorder

1. Don't Call Me a Hoarder: Carolina's Story 1
2. I Feel Guilty and Ashamed: LuAnn 11
3. Married to the Hoard: Isaac 17
4. Jessie's Inheritance 25
5. To the Outside World: A Professional Organizer's Perspective 31

Part 2. Understanding Hoarding Disorder

6. I'm Saving This Because… 35
7. Stuff or Overstuffed: Clutter, Collecting, Chronic Disorganization, and Hoarding 43
8. Is Hoarding a Compulsion or Addiction
   Insights from Marla W. Deibler, PsyD 53
9. Demystifying Hoarding Disorder and the *DSM-5*
   Michael Tompkins, PhD 61

Part 3. Successful Helping

10. Compassionate Helping and Understanding 75
11. Two Strategies: Demand Resistance
    with Susan Orenstein, PhD and Harm Reduction 81
12. It Takes a Community
    Tiffany deSilva, MSW, LSW, CPO-CD 87
13. Navigating in a Bowl of Alphabet Soup 97
14. Taking Out the Trash: When a Specialist Is Needed
    Christa López, A New Start Biorecovery 103
15. When You Call Metropolitan Organizing 109

Part 4. Where Do I Go From Here?

16. Resources 119

Foreword

Dedicated researchers, organizers, mental health professionals, public servants, help organizations, authors, and the media have increased public sensitivity to people encumbered by hoarding disorder. These intrepid helpers serve to release people from a hoarding process that intensifies when left behind closed doors. Families, friends, and neighbors of people who hoard seek methods to ease barriers to intervention and trust. People need support to make difficult choices when barriers seem impenetrable and lives are at risk. Some people with hoarding issues who have the courage and insight to face their internal obstacles want effective methods to improve their lives. Release from the enveloping hoarding process can invigorate lives by replacing objects with the richness of a direct connection with self and others.

The cost of hiding and ignoring this disorder goes far beyond the broken hearts and spirits, yet these are what most concern us. Geralin Thomas and the enlightening contributors to *From Hoarding to Hope: Understanding People Who Hoard and How to Help Them* share their years of experience and knowledge to reach a public awakened to the high prevalence and widespread effects of hoarding. They provide inroads to people cocooned by things and speak a no-nonsense, knowledgeable, and compassionate language unencumbered by stigma that offers hope for true healing and growth.

With Geralin Thomas's skill for making complex issues easy to understand, she presents content that is well-organized and accessible for specific concerns and inquiries. This book serves as a model for working together to assist the 2%-5% of our population with this disorder and the many other lives affected by it. Unique contributions from each author are unified by a common goal: to assist in transforming lives affected by hoarding. Geralin and her contributors give something back to people who seek help and the people who want to help them. This instrumental and enlightening book provides hope for valuable members of our community who would otherwise suffer the toll from a lifetime of hoarding disorder.

Suzanne Chabaud, PhD
Obsessive Compulsive Disorder Institute of Greater New Orleans

Introduction

Perhaps you are reading this book because you have watched television programs or documentaries on hoarding and want to know more. You may be reading this book because you are a service provider who seeks a better understanding of hoarding disorder. You may even have encountered hoarding disorder for the first time, and you feel helpless—yet you want to do *something*. I'm here to help you understand the total picture of hoarding disorder, also called hoarding: its origins, its effects on the person who hoards, and how it impacts those whose lives intersect with that person.

First, let's take a look at what *From Hoarding to Hope* is not:

It is not a diagnostic tool, with one exception. Dr. Michael Tompkins' chapter on hoarding disorder and the *DSM-5* is included primarily for behavioral health professionals and clinicians, because they are the only ones qualified and licensed to diagnose hoarding disorder. For the rest of us, however, it gives insight into the "inner workings" of making that diagnosis and the role insurance plans may or may not play in covering hoarding disorder.

It is not a professional organizer's list of tips or a professional organizer's textbook on how to work with someone with hoarding disorder or hoarding tendencies. However, *From Hoarding to Hope* gives you resources to consult for more information.

Second, let's take a look at what *From Hoarding to Hope* is:

It is a multidimensional approach to understanding hoarding disorder and hoarding tendencies.

It is a strategic guidebook, a starting point to help you assemble the right team should the need arise, perhaps for a loved one or as part of your job.

Third, here is what you will find in *From Hoarding to Hope:*

Part 1: The Face of Hoarding Disorder

Here, in *From Hoarding to Hope: Understanding People Who Hoard and How to Help Them*, you will meet some special people who originally shared their stories with me and my blog readers. It takes a lot of courage to share private struggles in a public forum. That they opened their homes and hearts to work with me as a professional organizer is a tremendous gift to me personally, but that they have willingly shared this freely is their gift to us all. Although we may be unable to walk in their shoes, let us, for a few moments, try to look at life through their eyes.

Caution: You may be disappointed if you are expecting a neatly wrapped story with a tidy ending as you might see in a documentary or on television. Remember that these vignettes capture a moment in time, not a lifetime of experiences. The positive side of this, however, is that we can come back to this "time bite" and bring ourselves into their story, really listening from the heart and reading between the lines. It is in these ways that I hope you will begin to develop compassion and understanding for the people and shift your focus away from the *stuff*.

Part 2: Understanding Hoarding Disorder

The second section looks at hoarding disorder/tendencies in the context of why we save stuff and the distinctions among clutter, collecting, chronic disorganization, and hoarding. Since I am often asked whether hoarding is a compulsion or an addiction, I included Dr. Marla Deibler's blog on that subject. Finally in this section, Dr. Michael Tompkins demystifies hoarding as an approved mental health diagnosis.

Part 3: Successful Helping

From Hoarding to Hope: Understanding People Who Hoard and How to Help Them explores the team approach to working with someone who hoards. It is a starting point—an introduction to the complex world of hoarding. It takes a community—a team—to help someone with hoarding disorder. If you watched television programs like *Hoarders* or *Hoarding: Buried Alive*, you will always see that team. The mental health clinician provides support. The professional organizer (often a team of them) helps clear the clutter. And, of course, the disposal company removes the debris. Also on the scene may be family members and friends who hopefully offer help and encouragement. Public health, law enforcement, fire and safety, great contractors and handymen, and animal control officials also may have been called to assist.

Part 4: Where Do I Go From Here?

The Internet provides us with virtually ever-changing, real-time information that is impossible to keep current in a book like this. *From Hoarding to Hope: Understanding People Who Hoard and How to Help Them* gives you a starting point. As you traverse the Internet, you can refine your searches to those that best fit your needs and situation.

Chapter 1

Don't Call Me a Hoarder: Carolina's Story

Perhaps one of most difficult cultural and societal challenges we encounter is stereotyping. The labels we apply to ourselves can become a self-fulfilling prophecy. For example, a child with an undiagnosed learning disability may experience failure upon failure and develop a self-image that proclaims "I am a failure." We unwittingly become what we believe, so we live out that truth as our reality.

What happens, however, when our perceived truth is altered? What occurs when a child's learning disability is diagnosed and an individualized learning plan is developed and implemented? The child "experiences" or "achieves" success and finally begins to see beyond the challenge to the potential that has been inside all along. The child discovers what we all know: Success breeds success.

This same kind of mindset-reframing is essential for all of us in order to transform our lives from any damaging self-labeling we have inflicted to embracing a self-image that helps us move forward. It's not easy, and sometimes those around us make it even more difficult. We may not be able to change the story that's already been written, but we can change the ending.

The Backstory

As a professional organizer, I know that clutter is never simply about the stuff; there is always a story behind it. For me, hearing someone's story is the best part of my job. As I listen, I pay attention to what the person says and how they say it. Equally important, I listen for what is *not* being said.

Television programs cannot capture the full story about the hoarding situation they are filming. It simply isn't possible. During the viewing hour, we peer into a very small corner of that story, but we cannot begin to understand *that person*—their thoughts, feelings, and experiences. *From Hoarding to Hope: Understanding People Who Hoard and How to Help Them* will help us connect a real face to a real story.

Carolina's Story

One of my clients generously agreed to share her story as a post on my blog several years ago and again on a follow-up blog post a couple of years later. I am very proud of all that she has accomplished and commend her for the hard work she has done. I hope her story gives you some insight into yourself or someone you know who may be struggling with organizational challenges.

Background

Carolina is 44 years old and widowed. She has a college degree in business administration and is an environmentalist and activist. Carolina enjoys bird-watching, volunteering, crafting, and viewing documentaries.

GERALIN:

Do you consider yourself to be someone who hoards? How long have you been collecting and saving?

CAROLINA:

I am chronically disorganized, not a hoarder. I don't really collect or save anything. I simply don't know how to sort, organize, and store what I have.

GERALIN:

Everyone has a story; what is yours?

CAROLINA:

I had to deal with becoming a widow at the age of 25. My husband was killed by a drunk driver in 1990. I then had a series of traumatic events during 1999-2001 and suffered a physical ailment that left me handicapped.

In the span of two and a half years, I lost both parents, my grandmother, my only uncle, a close friend, and all three of my pets. The grief was overwhelming. First came the aftershock from so many traumatic events so close together, and then depression. It took several years to work through the grief.

I put my deceased family members' belongings in my home (stuffed in every available nook and cranny). I literally put myself in a cocoon of stuff and shut out the world so that I could not only begin to heal emotionally but also learn to deal with a new physical handicap and limited mobility.

At first, all of the items stored in my home gave me comfort—each item gave me a tangible memory of all that I had lost. I wanted to hold on to everything for dear life after losing so much so quickly. Sometimes I would pass the time by shopping online. Because of the handicap, I could not go to the mall, grocery store, or department stores. Strolling through the virtual world online was easy and entertaining. Although I never had any sort of shopping addiction, the problem was that I was not getting rid of anything, just bringing in more stuff.

GERALIN:

How did you acquire most of the stuff that you've recently let go of?

CAROLINA:

I've always believed in quality over quantity, but I lost my way somewhere in this journey. I acquired much of my stuff by inheriting items from several different households of loved ones who passed away.

To help understand, let me back up a little. In September of 1997, my world was turned upside down when mom was diagnosed with lung and brain cancer. She underwent many treatments of chemotherapy and radiation, and the cancer went into remission. I had always been an avid traveler, but I stayed home with Mom while she was being treated. By March of 1999, I felt comfortable enough with her remission to make a trip to one of my favorite places—Alaska. While in Alaska, I contracted a MRSA infection in the form of necrotizing fasciitis (commonly known as flesh-eating bacteria) in my right foot and ankle. I was flown home, hospitalized for two weeks, underwent several surgeries, was in a wheelchair for two months, and had physical therapy for six months. I sustained permanent damage to the cartilage in my foot and ankle, which left me with limited mobility due to painful walking and standing. Mom took such great care of me while I was sick and in recovery—she stayed with me day and night and twice daily changed my wound dressings for three months. After six months, I was finally able to return to work. I had been back at work for only one week when we learned her cancer had returned, so I quit my job to help take care of her. Despite more chemotherapy and aggressive radiation, my mom passed away nine months later.

My father passed away only four and a half months after my mother, so it was a quick double blow, and in the next two years I lost others close to me as well.

Several years later, when I was finally at a point of being able to let go of some of their things, I had too much physical difficulty sorting, moving, and carrying things, so the cycle of living with clutter began.

GERALIN:

Since we began decluttering, what has shifted?

CAROLINA:

With the help from the Metropolitan Organizing team, I discovered that letting go of the "stuff" has made more room for the treasured items that have true sentimental value. I've learned to appreciate my things in a new way.

GERALIN:

What motivated you to ask for help?

CAROLINA:

About two to three years ago, I reached the point of not being able to stand the clutter. It was just all too much. I tried and failed many times attempting to attack the clutter myself, but it was too physically and emotionally draining. It felt like I was in a deep hole. I obsessed over what didn't get done. My frustration became resentment, and eventually I chose to do nothing rather than continuing to try. I expected to fail…and I did.

I became interested in a show on A&E called *Hoarders*. I was fascinated not only by the mental anguish these people suffered but also by the conditions in which they lived.

I realized that although I didn't live in squalor nor did I hoard by the clinical definition, I clearly had an issue with clutter. Furthermore, I learned that I could reach out for the help that I so desperately needed and wanted.

Until *Hoarders,* I didn't realize there was a specialty of professional organizers who worked with those who hoard. I knew there were organizers who would come straighten out a messy closet, but organize an entire house? Who knew?! When I heard the term "chronically disorganized," I said, "Hey, that's me!" A new world was about to open for me when I hit "send" on an email to Geralin Thomas. After watching her help others on the A&E's *Hoarder* series, I knew that a brand-new, shiny, organized world was a possibility for me.

GERALIN:

Is it stressful or tiring having organizers go through your belongings?

CAROLINA:

No, just the opposite—they are very helpful. They work quickly and know exactly how to categorize and sort items for me to go through. It makes the work less intense by easily identifying what is sentimental and what is just "stuff." It is a freeing and exhilarating process!

GERALIN:

What is the worst part about the cleanup process?

CAROLINA:

Sometimes it's hard to see the forest for the trees when everything in an entire room is pulled out to sort. It's visually overwhelming, but the organizer helps and supports me however I need it every step of the way. There aren't very many things I would classify as unpleasant about this process…except for the dust we stir up!

I realize everyone has a different background or situation that caused their hoarding or chronic disorganization. I am answering these questions from my own experiences in the hope that a reader who is looking for hope and help will find it here.

GERALIN:

What were you like as a kid?

CAROLINA:

I was always a responsible and well-mannered child. I made good grades, had nice friends, rarely disobeyed my parents and never caused trouble. I was the typical "good kid."

I've *always* been a messy person, even as a child. Occasionally Mom would get fed up with my messy room and clean/organize it while I was at school. My mother was very organized, and the house was always immaculate. She picked up after me on a daily basis, so in hindsight I realize that I never learned the basic skills of organization. But I don't blame my chronic disorganization on my mother—I should have figured it out for myself when I began living on my own.

Perfectionism is a problematic trait that I've always had, though you wouldn't think it if you had visited my house during the last few years. Typically, I will not do a project (or buy something) if it is not exactly as I want it. Most of the time I want it perfect or not at all—there are no gray areas or in-between. I am trying to learn to let go of these unrealistic expectations I put on myself and those around me.

GERALIN:

What is your most treasured item?

CAROLINA:

If I had an emergency, I would grab my two pets, a photo of

Mom and Dad, a book Mom wrote for me, and the pin collection from my travels.

GERALIN:

If you could have one wish come true for your home or life, what would it be?

CAROLINA:

I feel like I have come so far, and I'm proud of what I've accomplished. My dream would be to have a popular celebrity designer help me finish the process by turning my house into a home. I admire designers who can unleash their imaginative style to transform an ordinary house into a place of comfort, peace, and tranquility.

Editor's note: This story moved so many readers to request a follow-up "progress note" that my client agreed to share what happened next.

The Next Chapter

I am SO happy with how many [of your] readers are interested in my progress! (Thank you, all.) There has been a lot of progress since the original post.

I have settled in and developed my own maintenance routine. I know it's a learning process, and I do the "pick up and put away" whenever the mood strikes me, since cleanup is a quick ten-minute process. (Nearly instant gratification!)

Things look just as good as when the organizers finished. Having the housekeepers come every other week gives me immense satisfaction. My favorite things are getting into a sparkly clean bathtub, seeing all the vacuum streaks in the carpet, and having someone help me change the bed linens.

I've had a plumber, electrician, and a contractor here doing various tasks. We have moved mountains!

Even my two kitties have become more social. We've had tons of people in and out of the house, and they are immune to all strangers except the yardman. One of my cats, Bailey, despises the yardman because of the leaf blower!

I am going through a gazillion photos, and it is way more time-consuming than I expected. I'm editing (or pruning) though! I've kept roughly a third of what I've been through so far—the rest went into the shredder. Really, how many photos does one person need?

I look at the before photos, cringe, and think, "That's not me!" I have trouble remembering living that way because I didn't let it define me as a person despite being surrounded and crowded by STUFF. I had no idea how desperate I was until the process was finished. In hindsight, living with the clutter was more brutal than getting rid of it. Physical clutter = mental clutter.

Now that the house is decluttered and organized, it's a relief. That familiar feeling of desperation is long gone. However, I must confess, the process of sorting, editing, cleaning, and organizing was very hard work despite my being 100% committed to the process. (Anyone considering a project like this needs to be committed because it requires maximum mental and physical effort—it's not easy.)

I've finally finished the grieving process. Getting organized and staying on top of things has changed my life more than you can imagine. It's a wonderful feeling!

In Perspective

A person's experience and backstory are important contributors to how they view and interact with the world around them. Many individuals who display symptoms of or tendencies toward hoarding disorder have suffered trauma of some kind. For

Carolina, a series of emotional events prevented her from living the life she wanted. In a short period of time, she experienced the unexpected and traumatic loss of her husband, the deaths her parents and other loved ones, and a severe illness—all of which proved too much to overcome alone.

Before working with someone who struggles with hoarding disorder or chronic disorganization, take some time to get to know him or her. As you build rapport, you'll most likely discover the root cause of their unhealthy, and sometimes harmful, habits. When you address the origin of a hoarding disorder, you begin the healing process.

Chapter 2

I Feel Guilty and Ashamed: LuAnn

Television programs and documentaries about hoarding have helped many people acknowledge their need for help and recognize that they can seek assistance with their own challenges. Many reach out after watching an episode that closely resembles their own experience. Sometimes seeing another person struggle with hoarding is enough to prompt a person to seek help.

LuAnn's Story: In Her Words

Sometime after seeing a show about hoarding, I realized I have a problem. The episode showed a woman who could only walk through her home by following a very narrow path. All the extra space was filled with stuff. I saw myself in that woman. I've seen therapists before, but they haven't helped.

As I watched the series [on hoarding], I had to take breaks. I felt overwhelmed at how similar my thoughts and feelings were to the people on the show. I kept thinking, *"Me, too!"* Then I started to feel ashamed. I looked around my apartment and realized how bad it was. I've never had a lot of friends, but it had been years since a friend had been over. I know my son is embarrassed to invite his friends into our home.

I have two siblings who also struggle with a lot of the same issues—not to the degree that it's dangerous to their health, but their homes are filled with piles of stuff, too. I've asked them for help getting organized, but they don't seem to see the problem. They think my apartment looks normal, because it's normal to them.

I buy a lot of stuff from infomercials and can't seem to throw anything away. I save things like old newspapers, and I don't even know why. The stuff just ends up stacked against the wall until the pile is as high as my shoulders. I feel a lot of emotion when I think of my possessions. Not just with family heirlooms, but with T-shirts and books.

I need help, but I don't know where to turn.

GERALIN:

If you don't mind my asking, what do you think would help you most? You mentioned you've seen therapists in the past; have you ever been diagnosed with something?

LUANN:

I've been diagnosed with ADD in the past. I've never been treated for it, but I feel depressed.

GERALIN:

Do you think about your things when you are out of the house?

LUANN:

Yes, I think of my things a lot.

GERALIN:

How do you acquire things? Stores? Yard sales? Curbside?

LUANN:

It depends. I shop online from eBay. My siblings like to give me stuff. If I find something I really like, I buy it in every color. I have a lot of books and clothes. I often can't find items, so I just buy more.

GERALIN:

Do you have any issues with your weight?

LUANN:

Yes, I've always struggled with my weight. I'm the heaviest I've ever been and can't seem to stop eating candy. My doctors have told me I'll become diabetic if I don't change my diet.

GERALIN:

Have you ever worked with an organizer?

LUANN:

No. I'd like to, but I'm not sure who to contact.

GERALIN:

Are you uncomfortable if you aren't surrounded by things?

LUANN:

I don't know. It's been so long since my home was clean that I don't know what that would feel like.

GERALIN:

Do you collect anything?

LUANN:

I collected books until my husband started to ask me about my credit card bills. I've cut back, but I still own a lot of books.

GERALIN:

Typically, there is a huge gap for individuals who hoard

between their intentions and their actions. Sounds like this is what you are experiencing; is that accurate?

LUANN:

I see myself in the people on the series [*Hoarders*]. There's so much I relate to, like the woman who can barely walk through her house or the man who holds onto old tools thinking he'll be able to sell them at a yard sale. I'll try to clean up, but I feel like I don't get anywhere or make any progress. I need help moving stuff, and I want some emotional support.

I want my son to be able to have friends over. I want my husband to be happy. I feel guilty and ashamed.

GERALIN:

I encourage you to let go of guilt because it's the most non-productive, time-wasting, and energy-draining emotion there is—second to jealousy. Use that energy to motivate and educate yourself about yourself.

Here are some other questions for you to consider:
- Are you hoping that the books you bought will be worth more than you paid for them someday? Do you consider yourself more of a collector or an investor?
- Is your anxiety medication working?
- Are you shopping online when stressed?
- For help, start by reading some of the free articles on stopping over shopping at Dr. April Benson's website www.shopaholicnomore.com.
- Another good resource for you is the Institute for Challenging Disorganization website. Take a look at its Clutter-Hoarding Scale™ and see where you would place yourself.

In Perspective

Many individuals who suffer from hoarding disorder pull away from social interactions with friends and family. They avoid people when possible and often don't allow anyone into their home. They struggle with guilt and shame and may fear the harsh words or ridicule of others, simply preferring to be at home with their "things."

For those in the process of overcoming hoarding disorder, it's important to include family and friends in the healing process. Everyone benefits from addressing and forgiving past mistakes. When damaged relationships are repaired, those who hoard can begin to build the support network they need to be successful in moving from hoarding to hope.

Chapter 3

Married to the Hoard: Isaac

Often the first people to seek help with hoarding disorder are the family and friends of the person who hoards. I've had many family members contact me and ask how to help. In television programs about hoarding, we sometimes get a glimpse of the family dynamics behind the scenes, and most of the time, this isn't pretty. What we usually *don't* see, however, is the long-term effect of the hoarding situation on the individual's loved ones.

The Backstory

After watching an episode on one of the programs on hoarding, Isaac contacted me asking for advice. He generously agreed to allow me to share his story and our conversation. Isaac's story gives us the family perspective *not* seen on TV. I hope that the advice I gave one viewer will be helpful to others in similar situations.

ISAAC:
One thing about the show that makes it hard for me to watch is the way it affects the people living with those who hoard. I

feel their pain the most as my wife hoards just like her siblings do. I'd say her siblings' cases are nearly as severe as those seen on the show.

We've been married over 20 years, and there are plenty of times when I wanted to leave or ask her to leave. She has improved (in part due to therapy) but not nearly enough for me, considering the length of time I've been living in this situation. I want us to move out of our small apartment, but I don't want to simply end up providing her with more space to hoard things. Just coming home every day is very depressing, and I am miserable.

I was wondering if you have any advice for people living with someone who hoards, or if you can recommend a website that offers suggestions?

GERALIN:

There is a site that provides an outlet for family members who want to chat with like-minded spouses, siblings, or children of hoarders. Children of Hoarders (childrenofhoarders.com) is a site where you will find understanding and be able to discuss your challenges openly.

I think the show [*Hoarders*] is so popular with viewers for the very reason you mention—the pain family members endure when the individual who hoards appears to value their stuff more than a spouse, children, or friendships. For most viewers, it's unbelievable. I've overheard people talking about the show, and they often say, "You have to see it and hear it to believe it."

I have a few questions for you. I'm wondering at what point would "enough be enough" from your perspective regarding your wife's hoarding. Do you think she will ever get better?

ISAAC:

Basically, I want to be able to get to things when I need them without leaning over a huge pile of boxes or bags of old newspapers. I would like to get rid of the clutter so I can clean and organize our home. In order to do that, I have to have fewer things so they all have a place to go. There's just too much of it, especially books. I don't expect things to be immaculate or sparkling. But I don't want giant piles of books leaning against every wall and stacked on every piece of furniture. I want to be able to have someone come in—even if it's just a repairman—without feeling ashamed. I would like room enough to spare so I feel like this is my home, too.

As to whether there's any chance she'll get better, she has improved over the last few years. Her siblings' hoarding issues are about as bad as the people on the show. My wife's hoarding isn't as severe, but it's enough to put strain on our marriage. The question is always with me: Will my wife stay at her present level, or will she go down the same path as her relatives?

She can't seem to throw things away. Nearly all our possessions are her stuff. I can only do so much. Some of our friends were shocked when they found out about my wife's hoarding. They were extremely critical and unsupportive—some even suggested I divorce her. Others either downplay the problem or enable my wife's behavior. I feel like I have no one to lean on.

Any thoughts you'd care to offer?

GERALIN:

How is she accumulating things—is she shopping for them online or in-store? Dumpster diving? Stealing? Passively acquiring? What type of budget is in place?

ISAAC:

She's constantly ordering more stuff through QVC and HSN. Over the years she's racked up thousands of dollars in credit card debt. I've confronted her about her shopping and spending habits, but nothing ever changes. She doesn't even use the products she orders; they just get lost in the piles of other junk.

I'd like to save up enough money to move out of our apartment and buy a small house, but I don't see how that's possible if my wife continues to hoard.

GERALIN:

If you closed your credit card accounts, would stuff still come into the house? If so, how?

ISAAC:

I don't think it would change anything. She'd still find a way to bring more stuff into the house, or her siblings would start giving her things.

GERALIN:

What are her peak accumulating times? Daytime? Evening? Weekends?

ISAAC:

Evenings.

GERALIN:

Here is a tough question for many to answer honestly, but would you say your wife is lazy or unmotivated? Lacks energy? Has a limited attention span?

ISAAC:

She works hard at her job, but she's lazy when she gets home. She has no motivation and doesn't want to do anything but watch TV.

Over the years, therapists and doctors have diagnosed her with multiple conditions, but it's never consistent. She's been prescribed medication, but refuses to take it.

GERALIN:

Is she "high functioning" to the public but not so much at home?

ISAAC:

Yes, I don't think anyone at her job would ever guess what our home looks like. She's held the same job for over five years and always receives positive reviews. It seems that she's able to function normally at work and do a good job but doesn't apply the same effort at home. It's like she lives two lives.

GERALIN:

What activities does she enjoy doing?

ISAAC:

She used to like to travel, but I'm unable to take more than a few days off of work at a time. I've encouraged her to save up and visit friends in Colorado, but she doesn't seem interested.

GERALIN:

Is she hooked on sugary drinks? Candy? Breads?

ISAAC:

Yes, she eats a very unhealthy diet with lots of sugar. She's pre-diabetic. Her doctors have warned her to clean up her diet, but she doesn't seem to care. I've tried to help her lose weight, but she just hides candy and sugary treats around the house. I've even caught her hiding in the bathroom eating a candy bar.

GERALIN:

Have you ever worked with an organizer (who works with individuals who hoard) or a psychologist (who has experience with hoarding disorder)?

ISAAC:

My wife has seen therapists off and on throughout our marriage. I have pretty good health insurance, so she's able to see any doctor she needs to. She'll go see a therapist once or twice and then never see him again. She doesn't seem to trust them enough to really open up about the hoarding. From what I can tell, the doctors she's seen don't seem to take her behavior seriously or view it as a problem. She's been prescribed medication, but either takes it sporadically or doesn't even have the prescription filled.

GERALIN:

Just an observation—I've noticed when working with people who hoard, often they *think/believe* they *cannot* change their habits. The process is very, very slow but most of them can do it (with help).

Isaac's Follow-up

Isaac contacted me a few months after his blog post was published with the following update:

Thought I would give you an update. My wife and I have begun to contact professional organizers in our area. She's agreed to see a therapist and get some help. I've decided to go to the therapist with her so we can try to work through our problems. Thank you for your help.

In Perspective

Hoarding disorder has long-term effects not only for the person who hoards, but also for his or her loved ones. Perhaps no one is affected more than the immediate family, especially the spouse. The story of Isaac gives us a rare, intimate perspective on how hoarding disorder strains relationships. As they say, no man is an island. Mending relationships and opening lines of communication among family members is a critical aspect of helping someone who hoards.

Chapter 4

Jessie's Inheritance

What about the children?

Once in a while, media representations of hoarding disorder show us snippets of children living in a hoarding situation and what's happening with them in the "now" of that moment. Rarely do we see the fallout and long-term effects of hoarding on an adult child of one who hoards. Is the child doomed to repeat history? Maybe. Maybe not. Even if the visible circle of hoarding disorder is disrupted in the next generation, there may still be an internal aftermath and struggle that others never see. But it's there. And the tape that replays over and over again may sound something like this: "If my mother [father] is [was] one of those people like you see on TV, what does that make me? Am I going to be like *that?*" Can you imagine living with that thought constantly in the back of your mind, always reminding you of what "could" happen?

Meet Jessie Sholl, author of the book *Dirty Secret: A Daughter Comes Clean About Her Mother's Compulsive Hoarding.*

The Backstory

Jessie's mom wasn't like other moms. When Jessie was in kindergarten, her mom might choose to spend an afternoon thrift store shopping—and forget to pick Jessie up from school. Fast forward to Jessie's adult life after her mom's diagnosis of cancer. Jessie returned to her hometown to help her divorced mom prepare for her upcoming surgery and get her affairs in order. Once again for Jessie, the truth of her mother's compulsive hoarding was impossible to ignore. How does this play out for Jessie today? How does Jessie perceive her future? Is there hope that she will not "become her mother"?

I am grateful to Jessie for sharing this vignette with us. The fact that this happened on New Year's Eve has an ironic significance, as you will learn at the end of the story.

Jessie's Inheritance—In Her Words

It's New Year's Eve, and I'm cleaning my apartment. I'm vacuuming, sweeping, mopping, and scrubbing. I'm straightening the bookshelves, making sure there's not a speck of dust lurking under the couch or behind a chair.

My apartment is easy to clean because it doesn't contain much; I like it that way. I've always been a minimalist—actually I'm beyond a minimalist. I get a thrill out of throwing things away. I've given away stereos, televisions, vintage love seats, bookcases. I can't find my diploma from graduate school, and I have a feeling it ended up in the garbage during one of my purges. I even love getting to the end of a bottle of shampoo or a tube of toothpaste. It's exciting to throw things into the recycling bin or the garbage. Whenever I buy a new article of clothing, I toss something else to make room. Getting rid of things is liberating. Invigorating.

And for a long time, I spent way too much energy trying to get my mother to agree with the way I choose to live my life. Because my mother is the opposite of me: My mother has a compulsion to hoard.

From what I've seen, children of those who hoard tend to go one of two ways: We become hoarders, or we veer in the opposite direction and become what I call "purgers." Since 85% of those who hoard can recall a first-degree relative they'd describe as a pack rat, there's clearly a genetic component to hoarding; still, among siblings with a hoarding parent, it's not uncommon for one person to become a clutterbug and the other a major minimalist. Perhaps in the first case, it's a genetic predisposition combined with a learned behavior, and in the second case, purgers like me are the result of a rejection of what *could* have become a learned behavior—whether that rejection is on a conscious level or not. In my case, it was years before I even made a connection between my mother's hoarding and my preference for a lack of stuff. And I don't think her hoarding is the only reason I'm a minimalist. It's also simply an aesthetic preference.

So, on a rational level, I know my apartment isn't cluttered or messy. Yet every time I have a guest coming over—especially if it's an overnight guest—I have a mini-panic attack and go ballistic on the cleaning.

I've been like this for as long as I can remember, but it's gotten even worse since my book, *Dirty Secret: A Daughter Comes Clean About Her Mother's Compulsive Hoarding*, came out. To be clear, this is the ONLY area of my life that wasn't vastly enhanced by spilling my secret, and it is a small price to pay for all of the remarkable improvements I've seen in my life and in my relationships since the book's publication.

My guest anxiety isn't unusual for a child of a hoarder. We call it "doorbell dread." It can occur the moment one's doorbell rings unexpectedly—which never happens to me because I live in New York City where random pop-ins are *extremely* rare—or it can happen in the days or hours before a guest is due to arrive. My version of doorbell dread goes like this: I look around the apartment, declare it a pigsty, snap at my undeserving husband—something along the lines of, "So-and-so is going to be here in two hours, and this place is a hellhole!" Then I snatch the broom and dustpan from the closet and frantically race around in search of concealed clusters of mess.

Which is precisely how I'm behaving on New Year's Eve, for two reasons: A friend is coming into town tomorrow and spending the night on our couch, and the next day—and this is the source of my REAL nervousness—my friend, Liz, who runs the ultra-fabulous blog *Homebodies*, is coming to my apartment to take pictures. Which she'll then post on her blog. As in, the Internet. As in anyone in the world can see photos of my apartment, and what if I overlooked a cluster of clutter or a smattering of dust? Because everyone knows now about my mother, they'll see the horrible mess in my apartment and say, "Aha! Jessie is on the road to becoming a hoarder! After all, it is genetic..."

Okay.

Calm.

There.

After some deep breaths and reassurance from my husband that our apartment looks "fine," I'm fine too.

People often ask me whether I'm afraid I'll start hoarding, whether my low tolerance for clutter and for stuff will evaporate after a trauma the way it often does with those who hoard.

And despite my doorbell dread, the answer is no. I'm not afraid of becoming someone who hoards. I'll allow that perhaps a certain genetic pattern lies in my DNA, but that doesn't mean I'm doomed.

And I have a feeling I'm not doomed to suffer from doorbell dread forever, either. I really do enjoy having people over. My husband and I have been giving more parties in the last year, and I genuinely like doing it.

On New Year's Day, when our houseguest arrives, we'll enjoy a quiet dinner and a nice bottle of wine. She'll sleep peacefully on our couch and in the morning compliment us on our cozy and clean apartment. We'll go for brunch and then a long walk. I'll hardly have time even for spot cleaning before Liz comes over to take photographs for *Homebodies*.

And you know what? It doesn't matter.

Through my own version of exposure therapy, my doorbell dread is beginning to disappear. I have a feeling that soon it will be gone.

In Perspective

Many of the children of those with hoarding disorder live with a fear of hoarding. To counteract that fear, they often go to extremes to maintain a clean, organized home with very few belongings. Rather than hoard items, they constantly remove clutter from their lives. For children who weren't allowed to have friends over to the house, the effect can be even stronger. Much like Jessie, they suffer from doorbell dread and fear others' judgments about the cleanliness of their homes.

As a professional organizer, I know there's no such thing as a perfectly organized house. The living rooms on the covers of glossy magazines aren't lived in—they're staged. It's important to find the balance between extreme hoarding and extreme minimalism.

Chapter 5

To the Outside World: A Professional Organizer's Perspective

For Those on the Outside

I have been asked by many about what it is like to work with someone who hoards. While each situation is unique, there are commonalities I can draw upon to share my experience as a professional organizer with you. Other professional organizers may work differently and have different experiences to relate. There is no "right" or "wrong" way to help someone who hoards. Please keep in mind, however, that no professional organizer is qualified to diagnose hoarding disorder; only qualified medical and behavioral health professionals can do that. We'll talk more about that later.

For now, I've chosen the five questions I'm most commonly asked about when working with people who hoard. As you read about my experience and strategies, remember that uppermost in my mind at all times is that hoarding is a mental health disorder. Like most mental health disorders—or physical disabilities for that matter—the disorder, disability, or hoarding tendency is a fraction of a whole person. It does not define someone, nor does it place a value on their role in society.

Is there a lot of pressure and drama in real life when working with clients who hoard?

No! When starting almost any job, there are trust issues and a "dating period," so things move a lot slower and less rhythmically until we've established a working relationship. People who have hoarding tendencies typically work more slowly than clients who don't have acquiring and discarding challenges.

And for the record, there's very little drama. Most of the time it's just the client and me working quietly together and sometimes team members (assistant organizers) working in other parts of the home sorting and categorizing.

I've never felt scared or "creeped out" when working with a client who lives in a hoarded home. Once in a while grossed out, but not creeped out. As a matter of fact, I find quite the opposite is true.

Many clients are lonely and crave conversation. Perhaps because it's been so long since they've had anyone in their homes, they are often gabby and inquisitive. They love (and I do mean *love*) sharing stories about their stuff.

More often than not, I'm reminded of their "outside self"— outside their homes, they are high-functioning, witty, wise, well-educated, and insightful. Many of the people I work with have a *fantastic* sense of humor! It's as if they lead a double life; it's fascinating.

What would I see/hear if I were in a home while you were working with someone?

If you were a "fly on the wall," you'd see that as the client and I excavate layers of stuff, we go back in time—lots of memories, lots of stories, and lots of history. You would hear some great stories!

Sometimes I feel like an archeologist when I'm working in a client's home. You might hear statements like, "Oh, damn! Those are the hot pants I wore in the '60s. I could stop traffic back then; plus my house was spotless! Look how skinny I was!" The male client may say: "That belonged to my mother, and I promised her I'd give it to the woman I love." I'd casually ask, "How in the world did it get stuck here, in the surplus of cans of green beans situated between your baby grand piano and your front door?" [Note: We are in a living room, and there are pallets of green beans under lumber, newspapers, academic books, dirty laundry, computer parts, ammo—you name it.] Ever so slowly, he would unravel the story of his ex-girlfriend.

How do you stop yourself from puking? Aren't some of those smells vile?

Absolutely! I admit that occasionally I have "hangover odors," meaning I can't stop smelling "it." It sort of lingers in my hair, on my skin, and in my clothes, but I'll share a trick—I rely on a brand of strong cough drops called *Fisherman's Friend*. I pop a couple in my mouth, put on a face mask, and try not to let any "house air" in my mask. The strong aroma of the cough drops keeps my air intake "minty fresh"—or a lot more minty fresh than the alternative! I also put essential oil drops in my mask, especially when opening a fridge that hasn't had electricity for years. I once had a client tell me that she found my grapefruit essential oil drops "offensive" smelling. Ditto for lime and lavender. She said my cedar oil drops "stank." It's interesting that the smell of citrus bothered her when she had rotten food, mold, and feces in her home.

Are there some people who are more likely to hoard than others?

I have no idea whether there's a genetic marker or not. In my experience, the people with hoarding tendencies who tend to *reach out for* and *accept* help more often than not work in helping and nurturing positions and professions—nurses, teachers, and professors. They are very caring people and tend to hang onto things, perhaps hoping to enrich the lives of others or to be needed and useful.

How in the world do you remain so calm in the middle of all that chaos?

Nothing will be accomplished if I'm being judgmental or impatient. It's my job to remain professional and focused. I feel compassion for clients, their families, their neighbors, and the communities in which they live.

In Perspective

As we have seen, there is always the human element to what is happening in a hoarding situation. It's not really about the "stuff" at all. The stories of Carolina, Isaac, LuAnn, and Jessie give us a glimpse of hoarding disorder that perhaps you haven't seen before. I hope that their courage in sharing their stories will give someone who is struggling with hoarding the courage to begin moving forward to face their challenges. Or if one of your loved ones is hoarding, maybe my perspective will help you with a mind shift that diffuses some of the anger and frustration you might be experiencing.

In the next two chapters, we are going to shift our focus a bit to a more "academic" understanding of clutter, chronic disorganization, and hoarding as understood by professional organizers—first from the inside and then the outside. Following that, renowned psychologist Michael Tompkins, PhD, gives us more of the "clinical" information about hoarding disorder based on its official acceptance as a mental health diagnosis.

Chapter 6

I'm Saving This Because...

We All Have "Stuff"

We all have stuff, and frankly, we all think our "stuff" is made up of things we use and need on a daily basis. However, very few of us live in homes containing only the bare essentials. Furthermore, almost everyone has at least a few extra items, but it's an amount that someone *else* might term as excess. In our mind, however, it's logical and normal that we should hold on to our stuff.

Many of us save baby clothes (long after the baby has gone off to college), Grandma's best dishes (even though we no longer serve formal meals), and dusty mementos of events we attended long ago (that was *us*, wasn't it?).

Others have closets or cabinets overflowing with extras: craft and art supplies, collectibles, papers—you name it. Holding on to some of these things may nurture us and provide sentimental satisfaction. Keeping other things may offer the hope of earning us extra cash. But in many cases, maintaining the extra stuff creates clutter that usurps our space, costs us money, and steals our serenity.

Breaking Up Is Hard to Do

I'm often asked why people have such a tough time getting rid of stuff. The answer isn't simple and also depends upon the individual.

It is important to understand that difficulty in letting go of possessions occurs along a spectrum—from those with extreme hoarding disorders to extreme neat freaks. In between we'll find those who may be chronically disorganized and those who just haven't quite gotten comfortable with the idea of decluttering the hall closet.

Why is it so difficult to let go of our stuff? The short answer is that humans are complex beings. The longer answer is that our values and thoughts shape us and our feelings about our stuff. Things we have learned growing up and decisions we have made as adults all factor into the "why" equation. Think about it: In all areas of our life, we hold concepts about the way that we think things *should* be and how people *should* behave. These concepts are maintained by our day-to-day thoughts and general values. Unfortunately, few of us have a crystal-clear view of the way things actually *are*. Our misconceptions can produce behaviors that may not serve us well, despite our best intentions.

Hoarding, then, is just another example of how our thoughts and values can be misguided and get us into a pickle. Many experts in the field who examine hoarding are sharing their findings. As a result, we are beginning to gain a better understanding of some commonly held misconceptions that contribute to this behavior. It is important to remember that hoarding is very complex, and the following principles are some of the factors to consider when analyzing hoarding behavior and working toward change.

What's the Value of…?

The reasons people save and purchase items can be summarized by noting the three types of values that individuals place on possessions. First, items are believed to have *instrumental* value and are purchased or saved because they are viewed as practical, useful items. Example: "I am going to save this butter container because it will be great for storing leftovers."

Second, possessions are seen as having *sentimental* value. This is when the individual attributes emotional meaning and attachment to an item, and their possessions are seen as extensions of themselves or a representation of others. Example: "I am going to save all of my old college papers, because if I get rid of them I might not remember the information that I learned and will thus lose my knowledge." Or "If I throw away my child's artwork, it means that I am throwing away my child."

Third, possessions can have *intrinsic* value. An item may not necessarily be useful or meaningful, but it is saved because it is believed to have some characteristic that makes it too valuable to be discarded. Example: "This shirt doesn't fit, and it isn't very meaningful, but I really like the color; besides, it still has the tags on it."

It is important to remember that most of us experience these three values in relation to our possessions. However, for people who hoard, these values are applied more generally and felt more intensely than we can comprehend. Because of these factors, the accompanying actions are continually repeated. The result is hundreds of saved plastic containers, papers, art projects, and unused items. When hoarding is severe, almost anything can have attributed value. This is where we might see squalor conditions.

I Was Just Thinking…

Truthfully, our values drive our thoughts, and our thoughts may include erroneous beliefs about the nature and meaning of our possessions. When I work with any of my clients, I acknowledge that almost everyone has some difficulty in letting go of things. I also explain that we get attached to ideas about who we are (or were, or will be) in relation to the things we hold onto. Comprehending why it's difficult to let go of our stuff is the first step toward understanding our behavior. Once we reach this understanding, we can make changes to both behavior and environment, and these changes can bring great satisfaction.

Why Do We Do What We Do?

In my professional experience, I've noticed that people fall into one (or more) of four categories when it comes to difficulty in letting go of their stuff: Sentimental Savers, Eco-Minded Savers, Value-Minded Savers, and Resourceful Savers. Each category offers a slightly different twist on why people hold onto stuff.

Sentimental Savers

These are the people who can't let go of the fifty-five photos of their child blowing out birthday candles—even the bad pictures such as the ones where a thumb obscures everything except the bottom of a toddler's chin. Other people believe they *should* have (and therefore *must* have) a sentimental attachment to an item based on the fact that someone they loved once owned it. It's as if the connection to that person will be lost if they no longer possess the item.

Eco-Minded Savers

Many collections and piles accumulate for people who are conscious of their role in protecting the environment. They feel a keen personal responsibility for saving the planet. For these people, it's difficult to discard an item by other methodology other than a "perfectly" earth-friendly manner. The eco-minded saver adheres to this principle even when the cost of holding onto items compromises their own home, relationships, health, or safety. While the intention to "save our planet" is noble, it may backfire on the eco-minded saver. If it evolves into hoarding, it may actually result in the destruction of their own personal environment.

Value-Minded Savers

Most of us want to think of ourselves as frugal, wise, and aware of the value of a dollar. However, value-minded savers believe that their soda bottle collections, quarters from all 50 states, or [fill-in-the-blanks] are worth a fortune or *will* be worth a fortune *someday*. For these people, there's an instinct to assign value to everything based on the perceived potential value of an item or collection of similar items. Because they once saw odd sculpture appraised as a valuable find on *Antiques Roadshow*, they've come to believe every odd sculpture is likely to have the same power to reward the owner.

Resourceful Savers

These savers believe that everything has secret potential. They are convinced they'll find uses for the ordinary, everyday objects that cross their paths. Whether it's a bag of wine bottle corks, a pile of dolls with missing limbs, or empty prescription pill bottles, resourceful savers believe that things should be saved because they have the potential to be repurposed and made useful again.

Whether these savers have the time, energy, or ability to put effort into repurposing the items is of little concern and is an often unrelated, unconsidered issue.

At one end of the spectrum are individuals who hoard. They hold on to an abundance of items while continuing to acquire more stuff. This inability to let go eventually crowds them out of their own homes and perhaps others out of their lives. At the opposite end of the saving spectrum, the impact may be less apparent. However, not being able to let go can still cost the resourceful saver time and money and may harm relationships.

In Perspective

Thinking about all of this stuff—our values, thoughts, and the many reasons it's difficult to get rid of stuff—may for some seem a bit overwhelming. It is important to understand and remember that life is meant to be lived to its fullest, work is meant to be done, and sometimes disorganization happens in the midst of all this. Even for the most organized among us, life can throw us the proverbial "curveballs" where we feel like a gigantic sinkhole has opened up and swallowed us whole. Any of those curveballs has the potential to throw our surroundings into disarray. Aging parents may need extra care at the same time that our children are leaving the nest. Illness—our own or a loved one's—may necessitate shifting our focus temporarily. Death may steal a loved one and take with it our energy and desire to resume our normal routine. Or perhaps we have become over-committed, and being organized has become a burden we cannot carry. It's important to realize that any of these situations can greatly affect our ability to stay organized. It's okay. Life happens. Above all, we must be gentle with ourselves.

Moving On

As I said earlier, understanding why we have difficulty letting go of our possessions is not simple. It's not the "stuff" but our relationship to it that causes problems. In our brief look at different kinds of savers, did you recognize a friend, family member, colleague, client, or yourself? Does it mean that someone can be destined to become a person who hoards? Not at all. Saving and collecting things occurs on a continuum. It is when the scale tips to the extreme end that a hoarding situation may occur.

There is more! In the next chapter, we talk about the difference between everyday clutter, collecting, hoarding, and chronic disorganization. Understanding these differences can help us address those conditions more effectively and aid us in bringing organization and peace into our lives. Hopefully, this knowledge also will help us to understand our friends or relatives who are challenged by hoarding.

Chapter 7

Stuff or Overstuffed?
Clutter, Collecting,
Chronic Disorganization, and Hoarding

Defining Clutter

Here's a riddle for you: What seems to mysteriously grow and multiply, disappear, and yet never goes away? Clutter! Yes, clutter. It can start with just one unopened envelope left on the counter. That starts the "round tuit" pile, the stuff you'll get to when you get "around to it." "Later" turns into "tomorrow," and "tomorrow" turns into "next week". All the while, your "round tuit" pile grows. You don't notice this phenomenon because you are absorbed with other things. Maybe a month goes by. One day you notice that the available countertop real estate has totally or almost totally disappeared. How on earth did that pile of unopened mail get so big? Is it one of those mysteries of life? No. We simply become accustomed and desensitized to what is around us. Although our conscious mind doesn't consider it significant enough for us to take notice of the pile, our eyes and brain are continually processing these visual stimuli.

All of that subconscious processing *must* happen in order for us to navigate our environment safely. Can you imagine walking down the street and having to think about each step we take or consciously evaluate each and every object we encounter? How exhausting would that be? Similarly, a cluttered or disorganized environment can exhaust us. It's all the visual stimuli that our brains continually process. On one level, our environment may be disorganized or cluttered, but we become accustomed to the piles and choose to ignore them on a conscious level—that's how piles mysteriously disappear from our consciousness.

But how do you define "clutter"? Is it the pile of newspapers that you trip over every day that doesn't seem to bother anyone else in your household? Is it the sink full of dirty dishes that drives your loved ones crazy but doesn't bother you in the least? Does a colleague's messy desk drive you to distraction—yet he seems to be able to find needed items or papers without any effort? The point is: Clutter means different things to different people. We each have tipping points and tolerance levels before our "clutter alarms" call us to action. We then launch into an organizing or cleaning frenzy that often sends those around us into "duck and cover" mode.

Here's how I define clutter: any item that is not being used, not being appreciated, is taking up space, and has been forgotten about. These criteria help us make the mental shift from our *relationship* with our stuff to the stuff itself when we are deciding what to keep, discard, or donate. Defining clutter this way serves us well whether we are making decisions on items currently in our homes or about those long-forgotten items packed away.

What we've been thinking about is basically ordinary, everyday clutter. Keep this in mind as we shift gears and consider hoarding.

Hoarding

Hoarding involves the physical activity of purchasing or acquiring unneeded items and bringing them into the home. Additionally, hoarding produces physical reactions such as nausea and shortness of breath brought on by the fear of not having enough. The same physical response can happen to someone who hoards when they try to let go of an item. Psychological and emotional issues also factor into the hoarding equation. The individual who hoards may project emotional attachments onto specific objects and feel driven by various motivations to acquire and save specific items. They may:

- See value in every item or in specific types of items
- Fear that losing a newspaper or magazine will cause them to lose important information
- Purchase items compulsively
- Be unable to prioritize not only their household items, but also aspects of their lives
- React with an intensifying range of defense mechanisms from humor to weeping to anger when faced with discarding possessions

Thus far we've talked about everyday clutter and hoarding in particular. As we explore collecting and hoarding, the differentiation may seem a bit blurry. To the untrained eye, what may appear to be a hoarding situation may actually be a large or unruly collection. Let's examine this more closely.

Is Collecting the Same as Hoarding?

I'm often asked to differentiate between people with hoarding disorders/tendencies and people with large or unruly collections. There may appear to be similarities between collecting and hoarding.

However, collectors and hoarders actually stand on opposite ends of a single spectrum. For those who are not professional organizers, the differences might be confusing. Understanding the difference between hoarding and collecting is imperative. That said, when is the line between collecting and hoarding crossed?

In essence, someone who hoards "gathers" all sorts of stuff. That gatherer, however, has likely crossed the threshold of collecting and marched right into the realm of hoarding when:

- Shopping behaviors and acquiring evolve to the gathering and maintenance of countless objects that carry no value to others.
- The mounting bric-a-brac begins to creep across all available space to cover beds, countertops, couches, or staircases.
- Any attempt at discarding the detritus causes pain.

At this point you may be wondering: If the line is so fine between collecting and hoarding, can or will someone who collects turn into someone who hoards? Before we think about that question, there are three characteristics that distinguish those who hoard from true collectors. It can be valuable to take a look at the way they:

- Perceive value
- Maintain functionality
- Express pride and joy

Let's take a look at each of these, all the while keeping in mind that each situation and individual is unique. Tempting as it may be, we cannot generalize.

Perceiving Value

Most collectors consider the monetary value of their collections to be, at least partly, motivation for ownership.

Collectors are usually able to classify, quantify, and articulate their knowledge of the various items in their collection.

People with hoarding disorder, however, tend to collect items that have little or no financial worth. Additionally, they perceive value according to personal interpretations that might seem arbitrary to others.

Visual or functional appeal may inspire collectors to begin collecting, but most collectors plan to sell items for a profit or when the opportunity presents itself. Collectors also often aspire to upgrade their collections—selling or trading items of lesser value to acquire objects that they (and other members of a collecting community) consider to be of superior value.

On the other hand, individuals who hoard discern value differently and are usually at odds with culturally accepted norms of valuation. They rarely accept money or are willing to trade the things they amass, and the value they place on objects is based on sentiment or other emotional attachments. For them, the idea of letting go or severing their relationships with possessions—even in exchange for money or something of similar financial value—is painful. Thus, those who hoard rarely sell things they "collect."

Maintaining Functionality

Perceived versus actual value is only part of the equation. The impact of possessions on someone's ability to live comfortably plays a large role in differentiating hoarding from collecting.

Just as there may not seem to be any rhyme or reason as to why someone who hoards keeps something, there's also generally no apparent logic to how things are grouped or where they are stored. The hoard—the mass of uncategorized possessions—takes over the living spaces to the point that the rooms can no longer be used for their intended purposes. You may have seen many examples on television of kitchens that can no longer be used to prepare meals or bedrooms that can no longer be used for sleeping because of hoarding.

Serious collectors, on the other hand, usually sequester their collections, both to confer status and prevent damage. A collector may have lots of a specific type of item—china teacups, Beanie Babies, or Neil Diamond posters—but can still prepare meals and eat in the kitchen, sleep unencumbered on the bed in the bedroom, bathe in the bathroom, and entertain in the living room. On the other hand, a person with a hoarding disorder/tendency may be sleeping in a chair or on the floor because the bed is piled high with stuff, making it inaccessible for normal use.

Despite the accumulation of items, collectors are able to lead engaging social lives. In lieu of surrounding themselves with friends and family, however, individuals who hoard will often withdraw behind a barricade of stuff. To outsiders, they do not appear to be suffering. However, many admit to feelings of shame and isolation.

Expressing Pride and Joy

Finally, there is a vast chasm between the degree of personal satisfaction and delight that collectors derive from their possessions and the emotions evoked from the accumulations of those with hoarding disorder.

A collector's pride in ownership is obvious in the way the collection is curated—new acquisitions are analyzed and categorized. Thought is given to how items will be blended into the pre-existing collection. Collectors proudly display their possessions, offer visitors tours of what they own, and are gratified by the interest others show in their collections.

When the subject of recent acquisitions comes up in conversation, a collector's eyes light up. They are eager to discuss the manner in which an item was acquired, its "official" value, and any plans for their object's future. Collectors often spend great effort and resources to create appealing displays to show their collections in the best light, both literally and figuratively.

People with hoarding disorders, however, experience shame related to the items they've amassed. They avoid visitors and evade discussion of what they've accrued. Individuals who hoard often keep the very existence of their acquisitions a secret. When pressed, they may exhibit anxiety when trying to discuss the items surrounding them.

Objects in a hoard are usually not arranged into categories, and there is generally no intention to display items so they can be appreciated by others or themselves. Acquiring and keeping items may give hoarders a sense of comfort but does not provide joy.

Can Collecting Turn Into Hoarding?

I don't think it is likely that a collector will become someone who hoards. Additionally, I don't know of anyone who suddenly turned to hoarding. In my experience, hoarding is a gradual process. The clients I've worked with have not filled their homes in a week or a month. It wasn't as if they went on a binge and suddenly started saving or acquiring thousands of things. It's usually a slow, trickling-in process, a drip-drip-drip of incoming *random* things. In some hoarding situations, I see themes, similar to that of a collector: copper mugs, silver star-shaped belt buckles, or painted, cast-iron doorstops, to name a few. But these types of things are mixed in with stuff that has little or no value. In the eyes of a person with a hoarding disorder, all of their items are equal in value.

To them, a free tourism brochure can be equally important as the photograph of their son's high school graduation.

What Do I Look For?

I'm not qualified to diagnose hoarding disorder. I'm often asked whether there are any red flags that pop up that may alert me to potential challenges I might face in working with clients amidst their mountains of stuff. There are four "whens" I look for that alert me to a possible hoarding situation:

- *When the client can't part with anything.* Typically someone with hoarding disorder will hang onto stuff for one of three reasons: sentimental value, instrumental value (it's useful), or intrinsic value (it's interesting, unusual, or pretty).
- *When the client values things over relationships.* Do you remember Isaac? He felt that all of his wife's stuff was crowding him out of their home, and he wanted enough space to feel like he belonged there, too.
- *When no one else values what the client collects.* True collectors can trade or sell their collectibles; there's a market for what they've acquired. This is not true of most people with hoarding disorders. Their stuff is valuable *only* to them, and more often than not is viewed as worthless by the average person.
- *When things aren't sorted and categorized.* Everything is jumbled and nothing has a "home." For example, I have seen personal care items kept next to the dog's leash, which is beside a stack of very old, soiled newspapers piled on top of a case of canned beans. Underneath all of those items is an address book the client had misplaced years before.

We have certainly taken a circuitous route to answer the original question: Is collecting the same as hoarding? In general, I do not think so. Because understanding the difference is important, let's recap the important points.

- *Perceiving value.* Does the collection have a real monetary value, or is the value in the "eye of the beholder" who cannot let go of the items?
- *Maintaining functionality.* Although some collectors cover every single inch of their space with their *collectibles*, are the living spaces still serving their intended functions? In other words, does the kitchen function as a kitchen?
- *Expressing pride and joy.* Collectors are eager to share their prized possessions, give you the grand tour, and their delight is obvious. Individuals who hoard, however, often keep the very existence of their acquisitions a secret. If pressured, they may even exhibit anxiety when trying to discuss the items surrounding them.

We cannot close this chapter quite yet. There is one more point along the "clutter spectrum" we need to take a look at: chronic disorganization. Sometimes it can look like a hoarding situation, but it is not.

Chronic Disorganization

A person with chronic disorganization has been disorganized most of his/her life, and efforts to become organized have ultimately failed. Chronic disorganization causes negative feelings or consequences on a daily or near-daily basis. You might hear them say, "I'm a slob. I've always been a slob." Although they don't finish the thought out loud, the last part of the thought is, "And I'll always be a slob." It is a self-condemning, defeatist mindset that spills into other areas of life.

While chronic disorganization may result in clutter and loss of living space, it is not the same as hoarding. Chronic disorganization also may lead to clutter in the office, time management issues, and to reactionary responses rather than long-term planning. Chronic disorganization may be a result of ADD/ADHD, a chronic pain condition, dementia, or other health problems. In today's society, chronic disorganization is also on the rise as a result of the inundation of social messages in all media extolling the value of consumption: Buy more and you will be happier.

People with chronic disorganization may:
- Have clutter, including paper, boxes, or bags stacked in the office or home, but they are agreeable to letting things go
- Always run late for commitments and appointments
- Try to organize, but just don't have the energy, time, or focus
- Spend the majority of their time reacting to the situation of the moment rather than planning ahead and managing their time accordingly.

Moving On

I am often asked, "Is hoarding an addiction or compulsion?" I have been also asked by well-meaning family members, "Why not remove the person from the hoarding situation, clean out the house, and then return them to a nice clean home?" It's just not that simple! While I appreciate the interest of family members and friends and their concern for their loved one, I recommend compassion in an effort to help without doing harm. Questions also arise such as: Should hoarding be treated like an addiction? Should it be treated like a compulsive disorder? These questions certainly deserve answers, and in the next chapter, Marla Deibler, PsyD, executive director of the Center for Emotional Health of Greater Philadelphia, addresses them for us.

Chapter 8

Is Hoarding a Compulsion or Addiction? Insights from Marla W. Deibler, PsyD

Compulsion vs. Addiction

The notion of compulsion has been likened to addiction, yet they are very different constructs. Let's take a look at what we know about the similarities and differences in order to answer the burning question of why someone can't clean a hoarder's home for him/her. For brevity's sake, let's look at the two behaviors in simplistic terms (although they are both quite complex).

Marla W. Deibler, PsyD is a clinical psychologist and the founder and executive director of the Center for Emotional Health of Greater Philadelphia, LLC (CEH). Dr. Deibler is a nationally recognized expert in anxiety disorders and obsessive-compulsive and related disorders, including OCD, trichotillomania, excoriation (skin picking) disorder, and hoarding disorder. Dr. Deibler currently serves on the board of directors of OCD-NJ, the New Jersey affiliate of the International OCD Foundation (IOCDF). She also serves as faculty of the Trichotillomania Learning Center's (TLC) Professional Training Institute (PTI). Dr. Deibler authors a blog, *Therapy That Works*, for PsychCentral.com, a leading online mental health resource. Dr. Deibler is a graduate of the Behavior Therapy Training Institute, the country's foremost OCD and related disorders training program sponsored by the IOCDF, held at Massachusetts General Hospital/Harvard Medical School. Dr. Deibler gained her formative clinical experiences at the National Institute of Mental Health (NIMH), the National Institutes of Health (NIH), Children's National Medical Center, and the Kennedy Krieger Institute at Johns Hopkins University Medical Center. She gained specialized behavior therapy experience in the treatment of obsessive-compulsive spectrum disorders at the nationally recognized Behavior Therapy Center of Greater Washington. Dr. Deibler served as a clinician at the National Center for Phobias, Anxiety, and Depression. She also served on the clinical faculty at Temple University Schools of Medicine and Allied Health as well as Temple University Children's Medical Center.

The (Not-So) Simple Definitions

First and foremost, the constructs of compulsion and addiction are different, but not mutually exclusive. A *compulsion* is defined as an intense urge to engage in a behavior (e.g., acquisition, avoidance of discarding). This behavior is typically enacted in order to reduce anxiety and distress or to avoid experiencing such anxiety or distress, although common use of the word simply refers to the urge. An *addiction* is a multifaceted term that is described historically as a neurobiological disorder that involves a repeated behavior (e.g., drug use) despite negative consequences, tolerance to the drug (i.e., increasing amounts are needed to achieve the desired effects), and the experience of physical withdrawal symptoms (e.g., increased heart rate, tremors, sweating, possible seizures). Some more recent models of addiction suggest that psychological dependence alone may constitute addiction (e.g., gambling, shopping); however, many argue that these difficulties are better accounted for by other means such as impulsivity, mood dysregulation, or other factors; thus, addiction continues to require withdrawal and physiological dependence as diagnostic criteria.

The Technical Stuff

In terms of how the two behaviors look neurologically, there is still much to learn about brain function and dysfunction in these problems, particularly in hoarding.

Prominent *hoarding* behavior in those who have been diagnosed with obsessive-compulsive disorder has shown greater activity in the bilateral ventromedial prefrontal cortex (VMPFC—emotion regulation); reduced glucose metabolism in the dorsal anterior cingulate cortex (cognitive, motor, and emotional processing and reward-based decision-making); and increased metabolism in the right sensorimotor cortex. Hoarding symptoms appear to be associated with dysfunction in the frontolimbic network. In *addiction*, neuroimaging has shown abnormal activity in the prefrontal cortical regions and the amygdala (stimulus-reward associations) as well as the nucleus accumbens (i.e., striatum neurons—reward). Addictive substances increase the level of synaptic dopamine (necessary for reward and reinforcement) in the nucleus accumbens and, in the case of opiates, act on the opioid receptors in this area. Synaptic plasticity in the nucleus accumbens and the dorsal striatum also contributes to drug-craving and drug-seeking behaviors.

Maintenance of the Behavior Itself

Addiction behavior (e.g., drug use) initially produces a rewarding pleasurable feeling or "high" (positive reinforcement), which is sought, although this pleasure often habituates. When these substances are used repeatedly, molecular changes occur in the brain that promote continued use (continued reinforcement), and it becomes increasingly difficult for the individual to control the behavior as they seek to achieve a "high." The behavior is then further maintained by the development of physical withdrawal symptoms when the drug use is stopped. Individuals then also continue the behavior to avoid experiencing withdrawal symptoms (negative reinforcement).

Hoarding behavior may be also maintained by positive reinforcement in that some individuals experience excitement as they find and acquire items; however, the behavior is more prominently maintained by negative reinforcement, in that the individual experiences great distress and anxiety when faced with having to decide the disposition of a possession. In other words, these individuals are able to relieve their distress by putting off making decisions about disposition or discarding items, which leads to increased clutter and continued avoidance of sorting and/or discarding items.

Treatment of the Disorders (Without the Complication of Co-occurring Disorders)

Addiction is typically treated by detoxification (i.e., the initial stage of purging the drug from the body while reducing withdrawal symptoms) and rehabilitation (i.e., may involve medication and/or behavioral therapy). Behavioral therapy helps individuals maintain motivation, develop coping skills to resist cravings, develop more adaptive behaviors in response to antecedents (behavior triggers), develop problem-solving skills, avoid drugs, and prevent relapse, in addition to improving communication skills and relationships. Cognitive-behavioral therapy has been demonstrated to be effective in the treatment of *compulsive hoarding*; it involves helping individuals change the way they think about and make decisions about their possessions in order to control their behavior and their emotional attachment to possessions. This process involves a thorough behavior assessment (to learn each individual's contributing factors); psychoeducation (to improve insight and knowledge of the disorder); exposure/response prevention (E/RP—for those who actively acquire, this involves exposing them to situations in which they have the opportunity to acquire, while having them refrain from acquiring. This may be difficult for them initially, but with repeated E/RP, they habituate, or get used to, the situation and their distress decreases); cognitive restructuring (helping them to identify the flaws/distortions in their thought processes and change them to more adaptive/accurate/positive thoughts); and excavation exposure (exposing them to the process of decluttering by sorting through their items while utilizing and practicing improved decision-making skills).

Why Not Remove Compulsive Hoarders From Their Home and Clean It Up for Them?

Is treating drug abuse as simple as taking drugs away from the abuser/user and forcing them to detox? No, of course not. Why? The individuals would be likely to do anything to obtain drugs and return to using because:

- They must manage the strong neurobiological dependence that influences drug-craving and drug-seeking that has developed.
- They have not developed the skills necessary to cope with cravings and environmental "triggers."
- They need to improve problem-solving skills or address other psychopathology and stressors that are common in substance abuse.
- This also would not address the person's motivation to change; without a desire to end addiction, treatment will inevitably fail.

Compulsive hoarding is no different. This is why we can't simply remove individuals who hoard from their home and clean the home for them. First of all, doing so has the potential to cause significant distress and interpersonal conflict. Because of the great value placed upon many of these hoarded possessions, disposing them without the individual's consent typically causes them to feel violated and distraught. Moreover, it is not at all certain to produce long-term change; the individuals will be likely to quickly re-acquire and clutter the home and will be more resistant to further help or intervention. Cleaning for them does not give them the opportunity to practice and learn important decision-making skills, learn the function that hoarding has served in their lives, and learn strategies to cope with their intense emotions. Exposure allows them to learn that the emotions they have been avoiding (by failing to make decisions about items or discarding) are tolerable and that the intensity of distress and anxiety decreases (habituates) as they continue to proceed through the process of decision-making and decluttering. Therefore, they must do it themselves in order to be able to achieve long-term success and maintain the cleanliness of the home.

Take-Home Messages
- Hoarding is not an addiction; it does not involve tolerance or physiological dependence, and if the behavior were to cease, there would be no physical withdrawal symptoms.
- Hoarding is primarily driven by the strong urge to reduce or avoid anxiety or distress, whereas drug addiction is primarily driven by a desire for a "high."
- Treatments of addiction and compulsive hoarding share commonalities, but differ significantly.
- Individuals who compulsively hoard must engage in the process of sorting through their possessions themselves in order to be able to achieve long-term behavioral change.
- There remains much more to be learned about hoarding behaviors and what function these behaviors serve.

In Perspective

We have examined a lot in these few pages! We have looked at the distinctions of clutter, hoarding, collecting, and chronic disorganization through the eyes of a professional organizer. Dr.

Marla Deibler helped answer the oft-asked questions about hoarding: Is it a compulsion or an addiction? Can't we simply remove the individual who hoards from the situation, clean it up while he or she is in rehab, and then return them home once the situation is cleaned up? Our understanding of what's going on is now much better than 10 years ago. However, it's not enough because there is now another aspect we need to understand.

As of March 2013, the American Psychiatric Association classified hoarding disorder as a mental illness and included it in the *Diagnostic and Statistical Manual of Mental Disorders*, fifth edition, also known as the *DSM-5*. This will shape how the medical community and insurance companies view and support those with hoarding disorder. It may (or may not) make services more available. Adding this understanding to the total picture of hoarding disorder enhances our ability to advocate for those who need it.

Moving On

In the next chapter, *Demystifying Hoarding Disorder and the DSM-5*, Michael Tompkins, PhD, helps us understand what the *DSM-5* is, how diagnoses qualify for inclusion, and how the American Psychiatric Association (publisher of the *DSM-5*) defines hoarding disorder. Dr. Tompkins also addresses questions we may have, such as:

Are there any psychological tests that can be done to diagnose hoarding disorder?

Does making hoarding disorder an official diagnosis mean that insurance companies *have* to include this diagnosis in their covered services? Does it mean that they will help pay for services such as a professional organizer to help someone who hoards?

Does HIPPA (the privacy laws) prevent family members from sharing with a clinician information about their loved one who hoards?

The bottom line of all of this is you need not fear hoarding disorder or shun those who struggle with it. Rather, take the knowledge and understanding you've gained through *From Hoarding to Hope* and confidently advocate for your loved one.

Chapter 9

Demystifying Hoarding Disorder and the DSM-5
Michael Tompkins, PhD

"Hoarding disorder" was accepted as a diagnosis and published in the *DSM-5* in 2013. Great! It sounds so official and technical! But what does it mean? How does knowing about the *DSM-5* help me help someone who hoards? Can we get a translation, please?

As a professional organizer with extensive experience in working in hoarding situations, these are some of the questions that I had after the *DSM-5* was published. I have no doubt that others have asked the same questions. Although I am not a clinician, even I am asked about the *DSM*. After working with Dr.

Michael A. Tompkins is co-director of the San Francisco Bay Area Center for Cognitive Therapy; assistant clinical professor at the University of California, Berkeley; and a Diplomate and Founding Fellow of the Academy of Cognitive Therapy. He is the author or co-author of numerous articles and chapters on cognitive-behavior therapy and related topics, including *Clinician's Guide to Severe Hoarding: A Harm Reduction Approach* (Springer, 2014). Dr. Tompkins serves on the advisory board of Magination Press, the children's press of the American Psychological Association, and is a member of the Association of Behavioral and Cognitive Therapies, the Academy of Cognitive Therapy, and the American Psychological Association.

His self-help book, *Digging Out: Helping Your Loved One Manage Clutter, Hoarding, and Compulsive Acquiring* (with Tamara L. Hartl) (New Harbinger, 2009) received a Self-Help Book of Merit Award from the Association for Behavioral and Cognitive Therapies. In 2013, he was awarded the Lifetime Achievement Award for excellence in innovation, treatment, and research in the field of hoarding and cluttering by the Mental Health Association of San Francisco.

Michael Tompkins on *Hoarders*, I knew that he would be the perfect candidate to contribute to *From Hoarding to Hope* and demystify the *DSM-5* for us. I am so happy and grateful that he graciously agreed.

This Q&A Buffet

Don't let the clinical and academic jargon scare you. Read the questions first, and then go to the answers that meet your needs. Should you need any of the information later, it is here. Also, Dr. Tompkins has cited many supporting references within his answers if you need additional information on a topic.

Following are the questions I posed to Dr. Tompkins. Take a look and see which are most helpful to you.

What *is* the *DSM*? Who writes it? Who approves what is included and/or removed from it?

The *DSM* is the short name of the *Diagnostic and Statistical Manual of Mental Disorders*. It is a publication of the American Psychiatric Association and is the standard classification system of mental disorders used by mental health professionals in the United States. The *DSM-5* is the fifth edition of the *DSM*.

In the case of the hoarding disorder (HD) diagnosis, a *DSM-5* HD subwork group on hoarding disorder reviewed the peer-reviewed research and literature, consulted with experts on the topic, and tested the clinical validity of the diagnostic criteria through a process whereby clinicians use the diagnostic criteria in routine clinical practice. Following this lengthy process, the HD subgroup included hoarding disorder as a diagnosis in the *DSM-5* and placed it under the broad umbrella of obsessive-compulsive spectrum disorders, which also includes conditions such as obsessive-compulsive disorder, body dysmorphic disorder, compulsive skin picking, and compulsive hair pulling (trichotillomania).

How does a diagnosis get included in the *DSM*?

A principal committee of the American Psychiatric Association, with recommendations from the subwork groups, decides which diagnoses to include.

What is the definition of hoarding disorder as it reads in the *DSM-5*?

The *DSM-5* criteria for hoarding disorder are based on the original operational definition of "compulsive hoarding" proposed 15 years ago by Frost and Hartl (1996). The *DSM-5* refined this definition to include six criteria:

- *Criterion A*: Persistent difficulty discarding or parting with possessions, regardless of their actual value
- *Criterion B*: This difficulty discarding or parting with possessions is due to a perceived need to save the items and to avoid the distress associated with discarding them.
- *Criterion C*: The difficulty discarding possessions results in the accumulation of possessions that congest and clutter active living areas and substantially compromise their intended use. If living areas are uncluttered, it is only because of the interventions of third parties (e.g., family members, cleaners, authorities).
- *Criterion D*: The hoarding causes clinically significant distress or impairment in social, occupational, or other important areas of functioning (including maintaining a safe environment for self and others).

- *Criterion E*: The hoarding is not attributable to another medical condition (e.g., brain injury, cerebrovascular disease, Prader-Willi Syndrome).
- *Criterion F*: The hoarding is not better accounted for because of the symptoms of another mental disorder (e.g., obsessions in obsessive-compulsive disorder, decreased energy in major depressive disorder, delusions in schizophrenia or another psychotic disorder, or cognitive deficits in major neurocognitive disorder e.g., restricted interests in autism spectrum disorder).

The *DSM-5* includes several *specifiers* that further clarify the course of a disorder, its severity, or special features of the disorder. For example, in the case of hoarding disorder, the old *DSM-IV* specifier was "with poor insight," which was black and white—either you had poor insight or not. The *DSM-5* allows for degrees of insight: 1) good or fair insight; 2) poor insight; 3) absent insight/delusional.

- With excessive acquisition: If difficulty discarding possessions is accompanied by excessive acquisition of items that are not needed or for which there is no available space.
- With good or fair insight, with poor insight, or with absent insight or delusions.

If hoarding was once covered under the umbrella of another diagnosis (obsessive-compulsive disorder), how is the decision made to make it a "stand-alone" diagnosis?

Anecdotally, many individuals who have sought help for hoarding behavior in the past left the office of their psychiatrist or therapist with a diagnosis of obsessive-compulsive disorder (OCD). This is consistent with the view of the majority of OCD experts who agree that hoarding is one of several potentially overlapping dimensions of OCD (Mataix-Cols, Pertusa, & Leckman, 2007). However, the relationship between OCD and compulsive hoarding has been the focus of considerable debate. Emerging research suggests that it may not be accurate to classify a hoarding problem as OCD.

Researchers historically have presumed hoarding to be associated with OCD for a couple of reasons, including its prevalence among individuals who have other OCD symptoms and its correlation with other obsessive-compulsive symptoms. First, studies examining the prevalence of hoarding symptoms among those with OCD suggest that the two conditions often occur together. The prevalence rate of hoarding symptoms among those with OCD is between 14% and 42% (Fontenelle, Mendlowicz, Soares, & Versiani, 2004; Frost, Krause, & Steketee, 1996; Rasmussen & Eisen, 1992; Samuels et al., 2002; Sobin et al., 2000). This means that there is a good chance that someone who has OCD also will display hoarding symptoms. However, the majority of those with OCD do not have hoarding behaviors (Frost Steketee, Tolin, & Brown, 2006), further indicating that hoarding symptoms often occur independently from OCD.

Furthermore, Wu and Watson (2005) found that the prevalence of hoarding behavior among OCD clients is not significantly higher than the prevalence of hoarding behavior among a mixed outpatient group or even among control subjects.

In fact, there is a host of disorders and problems that accompany hoarding symptoms, including dementia (Greenberg, Witzum, & Levy 1990; Hwang, Tsai, Yang, Liu, & Lirng 1998); post-traumatic stress disorder (PTSD; Cromer, Schmidt, & Murphy,

2007; Hartl et al., 2005); Attention Deficit/Hyperactivity Disorder (ADHD; Grisham, Brown, Savage, Steketee, & Barlow, 2007; Hartl et al., 2005); brain injury (Eslinger & Damasio, 1985); social phobia (Steketee, Frost, Wincze, Greene, & Douglass, 2000); and alcohol dependence (Samuels et al., 2008). Investigators also have found hoarding to co-occur with bipolar II disorder and eating disorders (Fontenelle, Mendlowicz, Soares, & Versiani, 2004; Frankenburg, 1984). Therefore, researchers could conceptualize hoarding much like they do depression—hoarding can accompany almost any other clinical presentation but remain its own disorder. OCD is likely just one of the many clinical problems in which hoarding behavior can appear.

The second link that hoarding has with OCD is its correlation with selected measures of obsessive-compulsive phenomena. Hoarding symptoms correlate with OCD symptoms and traits such as indecisiveness, perfectionism, responsibility, checking, and doubting in both clinical and nonclinical samples (Frost & Gross, 1993). This would suggest that hoarding and OCD-related phenomena are similar in nature. However, several recent studies indicate that hoarding symptoms do not correlate with OCD-related phenomena to the same extent that other traditional OCD constructs intercorrelate with one another.

For example, although hoarding correlates with checking, washing, and contamination symptoms on measures of OCD, the correlation is more modest than that among those three OC symptom domains with one another (Abramowitz, Wheaton, & Storch, 2008; Wu & Watson, 2005). Also, hoarding correlates almost as strongly with measures of general distress as it does with OCD. In that regard, there seems to be no special link between hoarding and OCD, per se.

Additional evidence that hoarding is distinct from OCD comes from factor and cluster analyses of hoarding symptoms. Investigators have identified a series of factors or clusters of typical OCD symptoms in which hoarding symptoms consistently separate out as independent or linked only to symmetry or ordering (Baer, 1994; Calamari, Wiegartz, & Janeck, 1999; Summerfeldt, Richter, Antony, & Swinson, 1999). Consistent with the findings of individual studies, a review of 12 factor-analytic studies of OCD yielded the four consistent factors of symmetry/ordering, hoarding, contamination/cleaning, and obsessions/checking (Mataix-Cols, Rosario-Campos, & Leckman, 2005). This suggests that hoarding typically emerges as independent from other OC symptoms.

Not only do hoarding symptoms appear to be distinct from other OC symptoms, but hoarding symptoms do not respond as well to the typical treatments for OCD. Specifically, hoarding symptoms in several studies predict poor response to those treatments that are generally effective for OCD, including medication (selective serotonin reuptake inhibitors) and cognitive behavioral therapy (Black et al., 1998; Mataix-Cols et al., 1999; Winsberg, et al., 1999). Furthermore, OCD clients who also have hoarding symptoms drop out of treatment prematurely when compared with their non-hoarding counterparts (Mataix-Cols, Marks, Greist, Kobak, & Baer, 2002). Results such as these suggest that typical treatments for OCD do not target the underlying psychobiological or pharmacological factors that influence hoarding symptoms. Investigators have speculated that neuroanatomical differences may reflect unique psychobiological underpinnings of compulsive hoarding. Neuroimaging studies reveal different patterns of brain metabolism between hoarding symptoms and other OCD symptoms (Mataix-Cols et al., 2004; Saxena et al., 2004).

In sum, recent investigations suggest that hoarding disorder is a syndrome that is clinically distinct from OCD (Rachman, Elliott, Shafran, & Radomsky, 2009). Therefore, researchers recently have concluded that it is best not to include hoarding among the varied symptoms of OCD (e.g., Abramowitz et al., 2008). Hoarding symptoms are present in a wide array of psychological and medical conditions and may look somewhat different depending on the pathology that maintains these other conditions. While some individuals with OCD have hoarding symptoms, Abramowitz and colleagues liken this relationship to that of substance abuse and PTSD: While many individuals with PTSD report substance abuse, substance abuse is not a symptom or sign of PTSD.

What diagnostic tests could a clinician use to determine if a client has hoarding disorder?

Psychiatric or psychological diagnoses are generally determined by a clinical interview accompanied by measures. For example, the Hoarding Rating Scale inventory (HRS-I) is composed of five descriptors intended to reflect the proposed dimensions of hoarding:

- Difficulty using living spaces due to clutter
- Difficulty discarding possessions
- Excessive acquisition of objects
- Emotional distress due to hoarding behaviors
- Functional impairment due to hoarding behaviors.

Each item is rated on a 9-point scale from 0 (none) to 9 (extreme). The interviewer asks the initial questions, probing with follow-up questions (based on clinician judgment) as needed to make an independent rating of severity.

Are clinicians also likely to use corroborating information such as talking with family members, reports from agencies, and even a visit to the individual's home to make a hoarding disorder diagnosis?

Yes, contact with family members, agencies, and others involved in the patient's care is very helpful. However, the patient can deny the clinician permission to contact these sources, and the clinician is ethically and legally bound to honor the patient's request. It is, however, essential that a clinician treating a patient with hoarding disorder visit the patient's home. In fact, hoarding disorder cannot be treated without in-home visits, including an in-home assessment. However, I do not advise the clinician to arrive at the patient's home without permission, and the clinician certainly cannot force his or her way into the patient's home. I advise full transparency regarding in-home visits and other aspects of the treatment plan.

HIPPA prohibits a clinician from discussing anything about an individual without express written consent. Can family members or others share information with a clinician about a person who they suspect may have a hoarding disorder?

Family members can provide information to a clinician without written consent of the patient; however, this is tricky because a clinician who even accepts a call implicitly breaks confidentiality by admitting the individual is a patient. Furthermore, I recommend the clinician inform the patient that the family has contacted him or her and ask the patient how to proceed. For example, if the family calls the clinician and leaves a message, the clinician could listen to the message (but not respond to the family member in any way); this does not breach confidentiality, but it can undermine the patient's trust in the clinician if the clinician withholds information from the patient. I recommend transparency at all times.

How does a new diagnosis work with insurance companies? If it's in the DSM-5, is insurance required to cover it, or can they pick and choose which conditions they will and will not cover?

Insurance companies must by law cover certain diagnoses in the *DSM*. These are referred to as parity diagnoses, at least in the state of California (AB 88) and some other states, such as Massachusetts, but I do not know whether all states have parity legislation. Parity diagnoses at this time include: anorexia nervosa, bipolar disorder, bulimia nervosa, major depression, obsessive-compulsive disorder, panic disorder, pervasive developmental disorder, schizoaffective disorder, and schizophrenia. Some insurance companies have started to include more diagnoses under the same terms as the parity diagnoses, although they are not technically protected by parity legislation. Although the term "parity" suggests that insurance companies will reimburse patients who received mental health services for these diagnoses in the same way that the company would for a medical diagnoses or illnesses, insurance companies may still reimburse mental health services for these diagnoses (medical, psychological) differently. Professional organizers who are not mental health providers cannot bill insurance companies for organizing services.

[Editor's note: Check with your insurance company for details of coverage. You will need to ask to speak with someone regarding behavioral or mental health and medical diagnoses. Be aware that these services may be outsourced to a different company other than the medical insurer. The back of the health insurance card often contains separate contact information for behavioral health questions.]

How will the new diagnosis of hoarding disorder work with disability agencies such as Medicare and Medicaid? If it's in the *DSM-5*, are these agencies required to cover it? Or can they pick and choose which conditions they will and will not cover?

Federal law may differ on this from state law parity legislation. However, the law may be different according to the Affordable Care Act.

What recommendations do you have for related professionals who might want to seek reimbursement from insurance companies for working with individuals with hoarding disorder? Clients often don't know whether their insurance will cover certain services. What's the process like working with insurance companies?

I am by no means an expert on this issue, but I would assume that insurance companies are not likely to reimburse certain professionals like organizers, particularly based on a mental health diagnosis. Insurance companies reimburse for treatment of mental and medical conditions. Related professionals would first have to make the case that mental health treatment is within the scope of practice of the profession and that the professional is qualified to diagnose and treat mental health conditions. I know that some professional organizers are licensed mental health providers. In that case, the insurance company may reimburse the organizer who bills for mental health services under his or her mental health license.

In Perspective

We have certainly covered a lot of ground in this section of *From Hoarding to Hope*. Just to jog your memory, we learned about:

- Why we acquire or save stuff and why it's hard to let go
- Clutter, collecting, chronic disorganization, and hoarding: how each is different, although they may appear to be similar
- Differentiating hoarding from a compulsion or addiction (thanks to Dr. Marla Deibler)
- Finally, Dr. Tompkins' most thorough answers to our questions offer the perfect wrap-up to round out our understanding of hoarding disorder.

Moving On

The logical questions now are: What do we do with all of this great information? How do we apply it? The final section of *From Hoarding to Hope* pulls it all together under the theme "Successful Helping"—the "how-to's" or the nuts and bolts of why we're learning about hoarding disorder in the first place!

Looking ahead, the topics in "Successful Helping" include:
- "Compassionate Helping and Understanding"
- "Demand Resistance" (Susan Orenstein, PhD) and "My Thoughts on Harm Reduction"
- "It Takes a Community" (Tiffany deSilva, MSW, LSW, CPO-CD)
- "Navigating in a Bowl of Alphabet Soup"
- "Taking Out the Trash: When a Specialist Is Needed" (Christa López from A New Start Biorecovery)
- "When to Call Metropolitan Organizing: What it's like to work with a professional organizer"

In the leadoff to our strategies for successfully working with a client, we look at compassionate helping and understanding. Compassion far surpasses feeling pity for someone. Compassion touches another at the heart level and extends itself for the good of another. It is the foundation upon which successful helping builds and succeeds.

Chapter 10

Compassionate Helping and Understanding

Unintentional Excavating

Sometimes I feel like an archeologist when I work with clients. As we work through the layers and layers of "stuff," the "whys" of all the stuff also surface. If you've ever helped a friend deal with any kind of problem, I'm sure you know what I mean. It's not that we intentionally set out to uncover past traumas, it just happens. Now what? Do we hurriedly grab our coats, say, "I've got to run," and then sprint out the door as fast as we can? I certainly hope not.

Hoarding Disorder From a Different Perspective

Remember, it's not about the "stuff"; it's about our relationship to the stuff. Recall the stories of Carolina, Isaac, Luann, and Jessie. They helped us put a face to hoarding disorder. But as we know, there is a person behind each face, a person who deserves the same care and respect as you and I do. Let's look at the human being underneath the hoard and how we can help.

Whether you are a family member, a friend of a loved one, a representative from a governmental agency required to intervene, a professional organizer, or a therapist, there is a common ground upon which we all stand in order for the intervention in a hoarding situation to be as successful as possible: compassionate helping and understanding.

Compassionate Helping

It does not require a college degree to bring compassion into any situation—hoarding included.

Sometimes compassionate help means that we are a sounding board for another. It simply requires shutting our mouths and actively listening to what is being said and what is *not* being said. The person may only need to experience the affirmation of being heard.

At other times, compassionate help means non-judgmentally observing what is happening in a person's life and gently suggesting that they may benefit from seeking the counsel of a trained professional.

If your friend has had a fever and a deep cough for a couple of weeks, you would suggest a visit to a physician out of loving concern. Does this make you a doctor? Of course not! Would that stop you from suggesting that someone seek medical help? Such obvious physical examples are easy to address. It's more difficult to talk about the damaging, destructive, or chronic behaviors or situations we observe, ones that can't be fixed by an antibiotic or rest. Nevertheless, when we care about someone and observe that his or her situation is unhealthy due to prolonged periods of deep unhappiness or a struggle with substance abuse, compassionate help is required.

Take action and voice your concern. Whether or not your suggestion is or acted on, compassionate help means that you "hang in there" with your friend or loved one because down the road they may decide you were right and seek the help needed.

Sometimes, however, compassionate helping may also mean "calling in the cavalry"—which could mean governmental agencies. Even if professionals are brought in, you can still consider yourself a compassionate helper by initiating the intervention.

Compassionate Understanding

Along with compassionate helping goes compassionate understanding. While it is similar to compassionate helping, compassionate understanding seeks to learn the root of a person's actions and is deeply concerned for their welfare and emotional health. Sometimes we glibly reply, "I know how you feel," when someone shares something very personal, such as a deep hurt that may have been festering for decades. The reality is that we can never experience the impact of a given situation on another person. An event that to us seems not so bad or even trivial might be so traumatic to another person that they actually experience post-traumatic stress disorder. For years.

Compassionate understanding, then, does not attempt to interject our feelings, emotions, or experiences into another's life. It does not attempt to solve a problem. It does not try to trivialize or explain away an issue. It does not mandate that the person forgive another or themselves. Rather, compassionate understanding means being present for a person, knowing that you are experiencing the privilege of being invited into the life of another where many others are not allowed. It's called "trust."

Forgiveness: An Essential Element of Compassion

Compassionate helping and understanding in a hoarding situation also requires us to consider the role of forgiveness. Search the Internet for "forgiveness," and you will find pages upon pages of references to consult. Important as forgiveness is, however, this book is not intended to cover the topic in depth. Rather, it is a starting point to help us be compassionate helpers.

Forgiveness and Letting Go

Bitterness and resentment are heavy burdens, often the result of traumatic or stressful experiences. When individuals hold grudges, they often feel like powerless victims. Grudges take up space in your mind and manifest as a constant black cloud, preventing you from living life to its fullest. Forgiveness can be a powerful tool because it fosters healing by allowing a person to empower himself and take control. Psychologists, life coaches, and spiritual leaders agree that the reason we forgive is not to excuse hurtful or heinous behavior. It's not about rekindling or establishing a relationship with the person who hurt you. Forgiveness is about an individual releasing the pain that an event or situation caused. It's about moving forward and letting go.

When traumatic or stressful experiences remain unaddressed, they can manifest themselves in many ways. People who were previously organized may find it difficult to maintain that level of organization during times of emotional distress such as transition due to illness or bereavement. Some people who hoard may need to forgive someone who has hurt them. Others may need to forgive themselves for allowing their situation to deteriorate. When dealing with a loved one's hoarding behavior, you may need to ask for forgiveness for the times you have not been supportive.

However, forgiveness is not a cure, nor can it be accomplished in a day. Forgiveness and the act of letting go is a process, one that is often long, slow, and painful.

If you feel the act of forgiveness would help you or a loved one heal from hoarding, I recommend that you seek the help of a spiritual leader or behavioral health professional. Choose the best fit for you. Look for individuals who have an approach that suits your circumstances and frame of reference.

If you are unable to meet one-on-one with a spiritual or secular expert, begin by reading books and blogs. Though this may not replace individualized care, it will provide you with a basic understanding of forgiveness and its role in overcoming hoarding disorder.

In Perspective

Understanding compassionate helping, compassionate understanding, and forgiveness is all well and good, but how do we put this into practice? How do we navigate around the "stuckness" of a situation? How do we let go of the desire for perfection? In other words, when is "good enough" good enough?

Moving On

In the next chapter, we explore two strategies: demand resistance and harm reduction. Susan Orenstein, PhD, talks about demand resistance, the unconscious negative response to demands, real or perceived, internal or external. This is where the judgmental "shoulda-coulda-woulda" factors into our compassionate helping equation. Understanding this is important for all who work with individuals who hoard because it helps us remove *our* expectations and fosters more compassionate helping and understanding. Similarly, harm reduction is a strategy that can enable us to be compassionate helpers. It offers a viable option to help the individual who hoards regain a safe environment without our expectation of what changes "should" occur.

Chapter 11

Demand Resistance: Insights From Susan Orenstein, PhD and My Thoughts on Harm Reduction

It's admirable to *want* to be a compassionate helper and a person who practices compassionate understanding. Understanding the judgmental "shoulda-coulda-woulda" mindset helps us understand why we dig our heels in, resisting the demands those judgments place on us. I am grateful for Dr. Orenstein's explanation and clarification of why this happens and her tips to help us get us unstuck from that perspective. Following her original post on my *Managing Modern Life* blog, I have included my own section on "harm reduction." Presenting demand resistance and harm reduction in tandem helps us understand and let go of preconceived ideas of which changes "should" happen in a hoarding situation and then reshape those ideas into what is actually best for the person we are trying to help.

Susan Orenstein, PhD, is a licensed psychologist and the founder of Orenstein Solutions P.A., a group practice with offices in Cary and Chapel Hill, NC. Here, she gives her perspective on demand resistance and hoarding.

Demand Resistance: Understanding It and Letting It Go
Dr. Orenstein

As a psychologist, I take great interest in the question of demand resistance, a fairly common psychological concept that isn't always identified. In simple terms, demand resistance is an *unconscious chronic negative response to demands, real or perceived, internal or external*. For example, "I really should clean up this room," or "Why should I clean to please other people?"

I remember early on in my marriage of 21 years, we had a tiff, and I said to my husband, "You're so stubborn!" He replied that I could have only perceived him as stubborn if I were being just as stubborn. Wow. That really made a lot of sense. We couldn't be in a tug of war if I wasn't also pulling on that rope. So whenever I can, I drop the rope and ask myself whether there's another approach I can take.

When you find you're in a tug of war with yourself or others—you're not reaching your goals or going at the pace that you'd like—my first recommendation would be to stop the resistance and let go of the proverbial rope.

Pondering how demand resistance leads to your "stuckness" (its sources, the causes) can be intriguing and fascinating, but unfortunately it won't help you get unstuck. When you're in quicksand, you don't have the luxury of taking time and energy to remember how you got there. Acknowledge that many patterns are longstanding, based on habits developed as children ("You're not the boss of me!"), but also have compassion for yourself and recognize that you're human and doing the best you can. Then, get out of the quicksand and onto a safe, peaceful shore.

In our private practice of solution-focused psychology, we feel it is more helpful to ask, "What's right with you?" instead of "What's wrong with you?" I draw a great deal of hope and inspiration from more positive psychology approaches that are present- and future-focused and foster resiliency. Working from the assumption that everyone has natural healing abilities, we help connect you to your strengths and resources and bypass demand resistance altogether.

Dr. Orenstein's Tips for Getting Unstuck
1. Recognize that you can change your behaviors before you change your thoughts and feelings. This may seem backward, yet it can work. You don't need to wait until the moment feels right to get started. Often once you get started, your motivation will kick in and create momentum for additional work.
2. Sit down with a sheet of paper and think of a time in your life when you've been productive, accomplished some goal, or overcome an obstacle. Identify the approach you took to handling this task, and ask yourself these questions:
    a. What were the steps that I took?
    b. Were there others who were there to support me?
    c. What beliefs did I have about myself that promoted my success?
    d. What other factors might have contributed to my ability to handle the situation?

Write down as much as you can about this situation, and use this memory as a road map for inspiration and guidance.
3. Make a difficult or tedious task more pleasant by enhancing your surroundings. Turn on some lively music, open the blinds to let in sunshine, wear your comfortable clothes, or make yourself a pot of coffee or tea.
4. After accomplishing a small goal, reward yourself with frequent fun breaks (check your email, pet your dog, work on a cross-

word puzzle, phone a friend, play a video game, or have a snack). Make sure you set a specific amount of time for work and for breaks so you don't get offtrack. For example, declutter a space for 25 minutes and then take a 15-minute break. Enjoy those breaks—you're working hard and deserve that downtime to recharge!

5. Hire a professional organizer to guide you, keep you on task, and provide you with ongoing support. They often have very good systems and strategies for sorting through your belongings, so take advantage of their expertise.

6. Seek out a therapist to help you get and stay on track. A therapist can help you set reasonable goals, believe in yourself, manage your stress, and overcome setbacks so you can be productive and feel good about yourself.

My Thoughts on Harm Reduction
Geralin Thomas

Is harm reduction a last resort or a place to start? Harm reduction is a strategy employed by many interventionists seeking an alternative approach to aid drug abusers. It offers an alternative approach to a standard problem. Using this method, interventionists are not attempting to cure the patient, client, or victim. Instead, they are trying to minimize the risks. An IV drug user, for example, would be given access to a fresh supply of clean needles as well as a means for disposing of dirty ones. This is done in lieu of attempting to stop the drug use entirely.

How then can harm reduction be applied to a hoarding situation when working with a professional organizer? The easiest way to explain this is to tell you about one of my clients.

Meet Grayson

Grayson's hoarding added a significant handicap to his life. Because the heat vents and access to his furnace were blocked, he was living in a cold house. When he contacted me and requested my organizing services, he clearly stated that he did not wish for me to help with his hoarding disorder. This was the perfect situation for me to implement the harm reduction method.

Grayson was not yet ready for change. He had spent years acquiring various articles and artifacts at flea markets and garage sales. The rooms of his house were full of his "treasures," packed floor-to-ceiling and with no spaces in between. Because of this, Grayson lived without heat for four years. He told me he couldn't take another winter without heat, so we mutually agreed that our collective goal would be to clear enough space around each vent so that air could flow back into the house.

However, the first step was to clear a path for the repairman to reach the heating unit. Its access was blocked by stacks of paper, old appliances, boxes of yard sale "treasures," and inherited furniture.

I knew Grayson wasn't ready to stop his hoarding or acquisition behaviors, nor was he ready to work with a therapist. He did, however, take what he considered to be a huge risk by allowing me into his home and showing me his living conditions. Rather than spending time, energy, and money discussing the root causes of his hoarding and the conditions and problems associated with it, we instead worked on curbing the downward spiral. I did not want to risk having him withdraw and isolate himself further, especially with another long, cold winter ahead. I believe it was the best use of my time and his resources to busy ourselves with moving things away from the vents so that we could then clear a path to the heating unit.

By giving Grayson ownership of his individual decisions, as well as the opportunity to deal with his most urgent problem—getting his home heated—we were able to focus on the implementation of a mutually agreeable strategy. I hoped that he would see me working *with* him, not against him, and decide that in the future we could safely and comfortably work together in his home to deal with additional issues caused by hoarding. That, however, was a choice he could make later. For now, we solved the problem of getting his home heated.

In Perspective

To recap: Carolina, Isaac, LuAnn, and Jessie helped us put a face to hoarding disorder. We've looked at clutter, collecting, chronic disorganization, and hoarding from an academic perspective. In my work as a professional organizer, I have learned the lessons of compassionate helping, compassionate understanding, and the role of forgiveness in working with someone who hoards.

Moving On

In this chapter, demand resistance and harm reduction showed us alternative approaches to achieve the outcome we might desire or expect from our clients or ourselves. Quite frankly, however, understanding all of this does not equip us to be effective compassionate helpers. It may mean that we need to "call in the cavalry"—government agencies, therapists, or professional organizers—to help in a hoarding situation. In the next chapter, Tiffany deSilva, MSW, LSW, CPO-CD, explains why this intervention is necessary and the circumstances that warrant it.

Chapter 12

It Takes a Community
Tiffany deSliva, MSW, LSW, CPO-CD

Professional organizers know that compulsive hoarding takes a toll not only on people who hoard, but on their families, friends, landlords, and neighbors, as well as all the public and private health and safety departments and agencies that ultimately become involved.

As Seen on TV

A common theme among many of the television programs or documentaries about hoarding is that intervention is necessitated by an emergency situation. There may be an imminent loss of a home or children if the hoarding is not remedied. The actual structure of a home may be compromised. Normal activities of daily living such as eating, bathing, and sleeping may be impossible because of the

---

Tiffany deSilva, MSW, LSW, CPO-CD, organizing and productivity coach and ADHD coach who has been featured on TLC's show *Hoarding: Buried Alive*, explained mandated reporting in a hoarding situation for my *Managing Modern Life* blog. She describes her background:" In addition to being a professional organizer, I am a licensed social worker. As such, I'm also a mandated reporter, which means I am required by law to report cases of abuse and neglect. Before working with my clients, I let them know that I uphold confidentiality except in cases I am required by law to report, or if there is a significant threat of harm or potential harm to them or someone else. This ensures my clients know exactly what to expect, as far as my confidentiality agreement is concerned."

hoard. Are the situations staged? Sadly, no. Do all hoarding situations require emergency intervention? Happily, no.

In Reality

Compulsive hoarding behaviors create serious safety concerns for individuals, their families, animals, and first responders like firefighters and police. Someone may fall, combustibles could ignite, and lack of access to entrances and exits poses a serious fire and health hazard if someone needs to enter or escape quickly. Insects and rodents feast on rotting foods, dust, and other debris. In addition, both humans and pets can become trapped or buried under piles.

In cases of compulsive hoarding, some or all of the following may occur:
- Social services departments become involved.
- The police are called in if there is a complaint filed by neighbors or family members.
- Property owners (if their tenant hoards) may need to deal with costly cleanup, animal control, and evictions. Legal costs are incurred if the individual is unable to live independently or make decisions.

Hoarding Task Forces

In order to respond to the many needs that arise from a hoarding situation, communities have formed interdisciplinary hoarding task forces involving representatives of agencies potentially needed to address the issue. Fairfax County in Virginia offers some history of how this can work.

Formed in 1998, the Fairfax County Residential Hoarding Task Force was the first of its kind. Officials from several county agencies realized that many were involved in trying to address hoarding situations from their varied areas of responsibility, but they were often acting independently and without a cohesive approach. The Hoarding Task Force changed all that. It combined the resources and expertise of multiple county agencies to provide a coordinated response to residential hoarding when it threatens life, safety, and property. This task force works to find solutions to each situation that benefit the resident, the community, and the county government.

To give you an idea of the agencies involved, below is the list of member agencies that are part of the Fairfax County Hoarding Task Force:

- Adult Protective Services and Child Protective Services
- Law Enforcement Services provided by the Police Department and Sheriff's Office
- Animal Services Division
- County Attorney's Office
- Fire and Rescue Department
- Health Department
- Department of Housing and Community Development
- Fairfax-Falls Church Community Services Board
- Mental Health Services
- Department of Planning and Zoning
- Department of Public Works and Environmental Services
- Office of Public Affairs
- Board of Supervisors.

Task Forces Experience Growth Nationally

Today, there are many hoarding task forces throughout the United States, although exact numbers are unknown. New ones are regularly being formed, not only in the U.S. but also in Canada and other countries. While the Fairfax County Task Force can be considered a model, each community ultimately brings together its own set of agencies and other responders, even if they do not have a formally organized task force. Contact your local or state government for more information in your area.

Mandated Reporting: When Exactly Can a Community Step In?

In 18 states and Puerto Rico, *anyone* who suspects abuse or neglect is required by law to report it, regardless of whether they are a county employee or simply a concerned neighbor. Canadian residents also are required by law to report child abuse or neglect. If you live in an area where reporting is not mandated by law, you can usually file a report anonymously. Check out www.childwelfare.gov for more information.

Crossing the Line

There are three types of cases in which hoarding crosses the line from being "harmless" clutter to a serious instance of neglect or self-neglect. These three scenarios are: hoarding involving animals; hoarding involving children; and hoarding involving vulnerable (e.g., disabled or dependent) or elderly adults.

Types of Neglect Associated With Hoarding
Animals

Hoarding involving animals often results in animal neglect. Animal neglect refers to the failure to provide adequate food and water, safe and sanitary shelter, veterinary care, socialization, and the opportunity to exercise. Animal neglect is associated with both hoarding of possessions and animal hoarding. Most of us can understand how difficult it might be to meet the basic needs of an animal living in a hoarding situation. Animal hoarding is often the most extreme form of animal neglect as it poses significant health hazards to the animals, to anyone living in the home, and even to neighboring households. However, someone who hoards animals may not realize or may refuse to believe that their situation qualifies as animal neglect.

Children and Vulnerable Adults

Hoarding involving children may result in child neglect if the hoarding is affecting the parents' ability to provide the children with basic needs such as food, water, clothing, or a safe and sanitary place to live. Similarly, neglect occurs when hoarding negatively impacts a caregiver's ability to meet the basic needs of an elderly or vulnerable adult. As described in animal hoarding above, the person who hoards may not realize or may refuse to believe that their hoarding behavior leads to neglect.

Adults

According to the Aging and Disability Services Administration, self-neglect occurs when a vulnerable adult fails to adequately provide for him- or herself and jeopardizes his or her well-being. This includes a vulnerable adult living in hazardous, unsafe, or unsanitary living conditions or not having adequate food or water. A cognitively or physically impaired adult living in a hoarded home would be an example of self-neglect. If the adult is of sound body and mind and *could* independently care for himself, it is *not* considered to be self-neglect.

Unsafe conditions in a hoarded home that may constitute neglect:
- Significant rodent or animal infestation
- Significant insect infestation, such as roaches, fleas, lice, bedbugs, and so forth

- Extreme disrepair of the home (broken windows, structural damage, etc.)
- Human and/or animal feces that is allowed to collect in the home in an unsanitary manner
- Diseased or dangerous pets (e.g., a dog with rabies)
- Animal hoarding
- Sharp or dangerous tools, objects, or weapons that are easily accessible to children
- Trash collecting on counters or spilling onto the floors
- Cluttered stairs or blocked exits
- Extensive clutter that impairs essential daily functions or creates a fire or safety hazard
- Fire hazards, such as improper wiring, improper use of extension cords, the inappropriate storage of combustibles or trash, and paper stored near the stove
- Significant mold in the home
- The presence of toxic chemicals, gases, or other substances (e.g., lead, asbestos, radon, or mercury)
- Lack of utilities such as heat, electricity, or running water

What You Can Do to Help

Below is my list of the top five things you can do to help someone in hoarding situations:

1. Create a plan for safety. Determine what the next steps are for restoring safety after you've discovered any health or safety hazards. Prioritize based on what is the most immediate threat. Wear a mask and protective clothing if necessary.
2. Focus on eliminating any existing safety or health hazards listed above. I recommend reading *Digging Out* by Dr. Michael A. Tompkins and Tamara L. Hartl to learn more about

harm reduction. If agencies are involved, they'll tell you what needs to be done to bring the home up to code or to restore safe conditions.

3. Find temporary safe shelter for children, vulnerable adults, elderly adults, or pets while you are working on eliminating the hazards in the home. Choices for temporary care include: shelters such as the Red Cross, staying with a relative, a hotel, respite care, adult daycare, or childcare centers.
4. Educate yourself on your area's local codes and laws regarding neglect. Agencies you might want to search for locally include: Child Protective Services (CPS), Adult Protective Services (APS), the health department, zoning and code enforcement, the Division of Fire/Fire Code Enforcement, and animal control. If you have a hoarding task force in your area, they may be able to direct you to other resources as well.
5. Bring in allies. Familiarize yourself with local agencies, businesses, and professionals that can help you. This is not a situation that you should handle on your own.

What to Do If There's a Stalemate

What do you do if you're working to help someone in a hoarding situation who is putting others or him- or herself (in the case of self-neglect) at risk and isn't making progress in clearing out the clutter? Or what if they aren't receptive to creating a safety plan? Under these circumstances, you will need to contact Child Protective Services, Adult Protective Services, or such an agency that is charged with looking out for those who cannot care for themselves.

If you do find yourself in a situation where you need to make a referral to Child Protective Services, Adult Protective

Services, or another agency, trust that you are doing the right thing to look out for those who are in danger and cannot be their own advocate. If you are a professional organizer, seek support from colleagues or other professionals to help you deal with the stress of making a referral. If you are a family member and you need to make a report, seek support from family, friends, colleagues, or professionals, and continue to support your relative who is struggling with hoarding.

If you are the person struggling with hoarding and you fear that you may be putting others at risk, reach out for help and work hard to eliminate any dangers. If agencies do get involved, try to remember that they are on your side. Their representatives want to help you ultimately recover, remain in your home, and keep your family intact. In situations where hoarding requires significant resources to re-create a safe environment, local agencies can be your biggest allies. As an organizer, making a referral is never easy, but it may be the necessary step for finally getting desperately needed help. Contacting an agency is never easy.

In Perspective

This chapter certainly presented the serious aspects of hoarding disorder. Although not all situations require heavy-duty, community-level intervention, it is good to know that there are resources available should the need arise. Above all, each of us who intervenes in any way in a hoarding situation needs to be acutely aware that we must do no harm. As I mentioned in the last chapter, if reducing that harm or potential to harm is the most we can do at that moment in time, it's a perfectly acceptable solution.

Moving On

It's good to know that services are available, but where can you go to ask for assistance? The next few chapters will help. I'll begin by helping you navigate the alphabet soup of professional credentials, which can be overwhelming and confusing. Next, I'll share how people contact me and the discernment process I use before stepping into someone's home. Finally, we'll examine the role of the disposal company. In a hoarding situation, there are often considerations beyond the normal clutter and trash cleanout, and Christa López (from A New Start Biorecovery) will show you why these specialists are an important part of the team. Rounding out this section on "Successful Helping" is the chapter "When You Call Metropolitan Organizing" (my company). My intent is to give those who have never called or used the services of a professional organizer a glimpse into how *I* approach a potential client who hoards. Other professional organizers may work differently, but at the very least it will give you a reference point to speak with them.

Chapter 13

Navigating in a Bowl of Alphabet Soup

Television programs about hoarding make it look so easy! The entire assembled team appears one morning at the client's home: professional organizer(s), a mental health professional, a disposal company, and anyone else they might need for a specific job. In three days, poof! They're finished and gone. The results: nothing short of miraculous.

Imagine All the People

Do you wonder how long it takes to realistically orchestrate a project like those you see on television? Approximately 20 hours are spent on calls to vendors, consultations, research, emails back and forth, detailed photo reviews, coordination of teams, shopping for products, etc. Travel time is not included. Let's take a look at the team we assembled to help Carolina:

- 3 professional organizers from Metropolitan Organizing; 2 for hands-on organizing and 1 for remote administrative duties
- 4 dear friends of the client to help with hands-on organizing
- 2 disposal trucks with 2 disposal workers per truck

- 4 house cleaners
- 1 carpet cleaner
- 1 power washer
- 1 handyman-friend and 1 licensed handyman
- 1 professional house painter
- 1 licensed exterminator
- Antique dealers/auction experts

Keep in mind, however, that your situation might be different—unless there is a court-ordered deadline to meet. You may end up contacting/contracting the same number of people, but you may not need to do it all at once. Thrown into your mix as well might be the need to find a mental health specialist (now called behavioral health) for counseling.

By this time, you might be thinking, "How do I find the right people—including a professional organizer—for my team? All those letters attached to a name. I feel like I'm trying to swim in a thick bowl of alphabet soup!"

Licensed or Certified: What's the Difference?

Briefly, when you are considering a behavioral health/mental health specialist, there is usually a state licensure involved. Professional organizers, on the other hand, are not licensed by a governmental agency, but many have special training and earned certification from the Board of Certified Professional Organizers or the Institute for Challenging Disorganization. Let's start with looking at licensed personnel.

License Required

Who can do what, and who is the best person for me? The first thing worth remembering is that there are several types of professionals qualified to help with mental health issues: psychiatrists, psychologists, social workers, professional counselors, and psychiatric nurses are the most common. In order to earn their degree(s), each type of professional has to complete specific training and licensing requirements before they are legally allowed to provide specific types of treatment.

The Psychologist: PhD and PsyD

While these doctors can offer specialized treatment for compulsive hoarding disorder/tendencies, they can't prescribe any medications. In most of the 50 states of the U.S., a psychologist must have completed a doctoral degree (like a PhD or PsyD) from a university program with specialized training and experience requirements, as well as successfully passed a licensure examination. Psychologists may offer psychotherapy and work with individuals, couples, families, and groups. Some psychologists are primarily involved with research, and others focus on teaching.

The Psychiatrist and Psychiatric Nurse: MD and APRN

Only a psychiatrist (MD) or psychiatric nurses in advanced practice (APRN, in most states) are qualified to prescribe medication.

A psychiatrist is a medical doctor (MD) who specializes in mental disorders, is licensed to practice medicine, and has completed a specified amount of training. Psychiatrists can evaluate and diagnose all types of mental disorders, provide medical treatments and psychotherapy, and work with psychological problems associated with medical disorders.

Psychiatric nurses are registered professional nurses who have advanced academic degrees at the master's level or above and are licensed to practice independently and provide primary mental health care services to individuals, families, groups, and communities.

More Degrees, Other Professionals

Check with your state board of licensure for details about which of these require a license to practice:

- The MSW or Clinical Social Worker (some states: Licensed Clinical Social Worker)
- The MFT or Marriage and Family Therapist (can also have an MFCC license)
- The LPC or Licensed Practicing Counselor (depending on the state licensure, they may be called a Licensed Mental Health Counselor—LMHC)
- The MA in Psychology or Master's Level Psychologist.

Professional Organizers

Some of the professional organizers you've seen on television are certified. (I earned a CPO-CD® in 2007.) Becoming certified requires many hours of training and actual hands-on experience. There are several types of credentialing paths available, but the two most well-known and respected are:

The Certified Professional Organizer (CPO®) certification is offered through the Board of Certification of Professional Organizers (BCPO). To become a CPO, the organizer must meet the requirements of professional experience and education and must pass a qualifying exam.

The Certified Professional Organizer in Chronic Disorganization (CPO-CD) certification is offered through the Institute for Challenging Disorganization (ICD). To become a CPO-CD, the organizer is required to complete an 18-month training program that focuses specifically on working with chronically disorganized clients, and then pass a peer review to earn this designation.

Why Two Certifications?

Professional organizers work with many different types of people on many different kinds of projects. Additionally, as discussed in Chapter Seven, there are many levels of disorganization. Becoming a Certified Professional Organizer (CPO) shows you've had experience working with many different types of clients, but it does *not* necessarily mean you've had experience working with clients who are chronically disorganized or suffer from compulsive hoarding.

Becoming a Certified Professional Organizer in Chronic Disorganization (CPO-CD®), however, means you have had a great deal of training and experience working with the chronically disorganized, as well as enough education to have a basic understanding of hoarding and what it takes to help someone who hoards. If you then choose to specialize in working with those who hoard, which I have done, you can obtain more training and education to more effectively help them.

Do You Need to Be Certified to Work With Those Who Hoard?

Many professional organizers are not certified; some of them are extremely experienced, and others are not. Certification is voluntary in this industry.

While you don't have to be certified to work as an organizer, it's strongly recommended that you have a lot of training and experience working with those who hoard in order to be truly helpful. If you have not spent time learning about hoarding and working one-on-one with this population, you risk doing more harm than good. At the very least, you would be wasting the client's time, energy, and money.

To learn more about professional organizing and the types of work we do and to find a professional organizer in your area, visit the National Association of Professional Organizers website, napo.net. Other resources for finding a professional organizer include: Professional Organizers in Canada (POC); the Australasian Association of Professional Organisers (AAPO); the Netherlands Professional Organizing Conference (NPOC); and the Japan Association of Life Organizers (JALO).

To learn more about chronic disorganization, explore online and print resources, and find professionals in your area, the Institute for Challenging Disorganization, challengingdisorganization.org, is a good resource.

In Perspective

It's time to climb out of the soup bowl and start interviewing people for your team. Interviewing? Yes, interviewing. It is imperative that each person you choose for your team is a good fit for your situation. There is a significant commitment of time and money required, and you want to make sure you get the best return on your investment. At the end of Chapter 16, there is a list of questions that you can use to speed up the interview process. Be sure to take good notes so you can make good choices!

Moving On

There is one service not included in this bowl of alphabet soup: Biorecovery Specialists—the people in hazmat suits you may have seen on television. Christa López of A New Start Biorecovery in Austin, Texas, explains this specialty in the next chapter.

Chapter 14

Taking Out the Trash: When a Specialist Is Needed
Christa López, A New Start Biorecovery

Biorecovery Specialists and Hoarding

When working with those who hoard, there are many people involved in the process. In addition to professional organizers, therapists, and junk removal teams, sometimes biorecovery specialists are needed too.

GERALIN:

Welcome, Christa. Would you please tell readers what biorecovery services include?

CHRISTA:

Removal of all biohazards through proper cleaning, disinfection, deodorization, and documented disposal of infectious materials, including the following:

- Trauma scenes
- Homicides

Christa López is the co-owner of New Start Biorecovery in Austin, Texas. She has been in the field for five years, trained as a biorecovery technician through the American Biorecovery Association, and has extensive related experience over the past 11+ years, which includes emergency services work and a master's degree in counseling.

- Suicides
- Crime scenes
- Decomposition
- Human/pet feces/waste
- Gross filth/hoarding/squalor
- Tear gas
- Medical waste/needle pickup
- Dead animals
- Industrial accidents
- Odor elimination
- Automobile biohazards
- Electrocutions

GERALIN:

Can we just use a regular cleaning or janitorial service to clean up blood or biohazardous waste?

CHRISTA:

If the residence has human/animal waste, poor air quality, medical waste, decomposing waste, biohazardous waste, or the like, it is imperative that a certified and well-trained company clean the residence. This is likely the case if the resident has left material lying about covered in blood, feces, etc., or if the resident is known to have an infectious disease such as hepatitis C or HIV/AIDS.

A local cleaning company is not equipped to tackle the level of cleaning needed under these circumstances. For example, if a homeowner lives on his/her own, has a staph infection, hoards, and has tissues, clothing, and bedding all about, the residence is all potentially covered in staph—including the walls, counters, bathrooms, and other hard surfaces—and a biorecovery company should be called.

GERALIN:

Do biorecovery companies counsel occupants, friends, families, and staff?

CHRISTA:

No. Biorecovery companies relieve owners, managers, co-workers, families, or friends from the physical hazards of cleaning the location of the incident. Biorecovery technicians should be professional in appearance and be very sensitive to the emotional needs of those affected by the situation, but they do not counsel.

GERALIN:

What training is involved to become a biorecovery technician?

CHRISTA:

First, the technician should be trained in blood-borne pathogens. This training can take place online because it does not involve any hands-on training.

Second, and most important, is obtaining biorecovery technician certification through the American Biorecovery Association.

Third, it is recommended that the individual shadow existing practitioners to learn the trade in a hands-on environment.

Important Questions to Ask

To know whom you are getting to clean a residence, ask about the company's certifications and trainings.

- How many years of experience does this company have?
- Where do they dispose of their biohazardous waste?
- Do they have positive references from past clients?
- Do they offer before and after photos of their work?
- Will they work with your insurance company, if applicable? (Insurance companies may work with certified technicians.)

These are just a few considerations in hiring the right company. Just remember, you get what you pay for. If you go with the lowest bid, you may not be getting what you expected or hoped for.

GERALIN:

What happens to bio-waste as opposed to regular waste—does disposing of it cost more?

CHRISTA:

Both storage and disposal of biohazardous waste is regulated by law. Disposal of medical waste/biohazardous waste in a landfill is against the law. Serious fines can be imposed if improper disposal is detected. It is more costly to dispose of regulated waste; however, the subsequent fines for improper disposal are not worth the risk of trying to skirt the law. Check out the laws pertaining to your situation by looking at local, state, and federal standards. Be sure to do your research!

GERALIN:

What other special services do biorecovery service providers recommend collaborating with when cleaning squalor/hoarding situations?

CHRISTA:

I'd recommend looking into licensed pest control and/or mold remediation, reputable air duct cleaning companies, and movers/storage companies.

Christa's Counsel on Biorecovery Specialists

For pest and air duct companies, ask about the products used in their work to be sure they are safe for the people, pets, and plants living in the home or residence.

Mold testing and remediation requires an individual who has been through extensive certification and licensing. It also requires individuals to obtain continuing education.

To be sure you get the right person for the job, check their certifications. Call a biorecovery technician and ask for referrals, or do your research through the Better Business Bureau, yelp.com, state licensing offices, or other recommending bodies. Even hiring a contractor to conduct rehab work requires research to make sure they are the best fit for the job.

Two of the most common and important fields of collaboration are with professional organizers and therapists. Both require confidentiality, in-depth training, and certification or licensing. Make sure that person has experience and knowledge of squalor/hoarder situations.

The best price doesn't always give the best product; remember that you get what you pay for and that exposure to biohazards and other hazardous waste is not an area where you should cut corners.

In Perspective

Having worked with professionals as described in the previous chapter, including biorecovery specialists like Christa López, I've come to realize that helping our clients is truly a team effort.

Moving On

I would be remiss if I did not include additional details involved in working with a professional organizer. Sometimes we are the first to be called by a person seeking help for hoarding. Other times, a therapist may initiate the call. Find out in the next chapter what happens when you call Metropolitan Organizing (my company).

Chapter 15

When You Call Metropolitan Organizing

If you watch a television program about hoarding, you may see a professional organizer magically appear on the scene to coordinate the team for that episode. Because of my work on *Hoarders*, I am often asked how people in "real life" find me. Also, with television programs as a reference point, they ask what they can expect if they work with me. I am very happy to share my experiences with you.

How Do Clients Find Me?
They usually contact me in one of three scenarios:
- The client may call me personally.
- A child (usually adult child) may call me about his/her family member—typically a parent.
- A therapist may refer a client to me.

When I Call, Do You Just Show Up?
Well, it doesn't quite work that way. Before I or any of my team go on site, I always have a nice, long chat with the caller—

usually about 30 to 45 minutes. I learned a long time ago that what is *not* being said is as important as what *is* and *how* it is being said. I typically start with very matter-of-fact questions to see if the caller has short, simple, matter-of-fact answers or long rambling responses. Many of the questions are the same in all three scenarios mentioned above, but there are differences. Imagine yourself as a fly on the wall in my office, and the following is what you might hear:

Client-Initiated Call
"I need to declutter, but I think I have a problem. What is the process?"

I answer, "Well, let's spend time talking about your home and maintenance of your home before we move into a conversation about clutter...are you agreeable, and if so, do you have time now?" Whether the conversation occurs at that time or later, the telephone interview follows the same sequence:

- How long have you lived in your current home?
- Who else lives with you, including pets and/or pests? [*My insight*: People usually laugh at this, and I get all sorts of clues from their humor—or lack of humor. I'm always pleasantly surprised by the number of folks who classify their kids/spouse as "pests," in a loving way, of course. I've even had people tell me about their encounters with head and pubic lice.]
- How many square feet is your home? [*My insight*: To my surprise, a lot of people have no idea how big their home is—not even a ballpark figure. Why is this important? If a person has no idea of the size of their home, chances are good that they may not realize that they do not have enough room for all their "stuff."]

- Can you send me a few photos of your kitchen, bathroom, and living room? [*My insight*: Most are okay with doing that, and it's true that a picture is worth a thousand words. In other words, does what they are telling me match the actual situation?]
- Could you describe how you are currently living in and using your home? [*My insight*: I'm looking for information about lifestyle here. "Well, I'm retired and rarely use my dining room and spare rooms anymore—once in a while, when my grandkids come from out of state to visit, but other than that, I love hanging out in my sunroom with my cats..." or, "I spend all day every day in my basement because I have a woodworking shop downstairs, and my wife is mad because my woodworking tools have taken over the basement, the steps leading to the basement, and the carport." Again, reading between the lines speaks volumes.]
- How many pets are in your home?
- How old are your pets? Who is their vet? [*My insight*: If they can't remember the name of the vet, I usually make a note of this, as it sometimes means they haven't been to the vet in a very long time—if ever.]
- When is the last time you had your home inspected for termites? Which company does your inspection?
- Have you had your home treated for silverfish, roaches, ants, or anything else in the last year? If so, which company are you contracted with?
- Do you have any type of help with cleaning, cooking, and landscaping your home on a continuing basis?
- Who is the last repair person you've had in your home? [*My insight*: Was it the cable guy, the HVAC person, or again, has it been *so* long that no one has been in?]

But it's not all about the environment; it's also about the person. The following questions focus more on the individual and may help make it clear whether or not a mental health professional should be involved.

- Is there a pending crisis or deadline that you must meet?
- What are your goals? Why are you seeking help? These can be really simple goals, but please be specific.
- Are you working with a therapist? Are you willing to work with a therapist?
- What made you decide to seek help (social worker, fire department, neighbors, landlord, or self-motivated)?
- Does your current home have staircases? A basement? A garage? An attic? Are they full?
- Do you have a storage unit? If so, how full is it? Do you have multiple storage units? What are the sizes?
- Can you cook and clean in your kitchen? Is the stove working? Do you have a microwave, and is it working? Can you use your sink? Do you have a dishwasher, and is it working?
- Do you shower in your bathroom? Sleep in your bed?
- Are you going through any transitions right now? Grief? Pregnancy? Divorce?
- What days and hours are you available to work on organizing-related tasks?
- Do you have a budget for this project?
- Are you obese or immobile?
- Do you have any health-related situations that I (the organizer) need to know about? Do you have trouble with shortness of breath, asthma, or any other physical health-related challenges that I need to know about when we work together?
- Do you have a history of anxiety disorders?

- Do you have pathways in your home?
- How high is your stuff: knee high, chest high, shoulder high, or above the head?

As you can see, these questions give a pretty good picture of the client's situation. Red flags might be raised by some of their answers, and there is a lot of information not verbalized that can be read "between the lines."

Family-Initiated Call

"My parents need to get help for their hoarding."

The same questions above apply, but there are a few more. In this situation, the call begins this way:

- Where do you live, and where do your parents live?
- Are you a minor—under 18?
- What types of things are being saved?
- Where/when are they acquiring things? Passive acquiring (hanging onto junk mail and plastic grocery bags)? Shopping (flea markets, thrift stores, online shopping, QVC, boutiques, and department stores)? Inheriting (furniture from relatives)?
- Do you think both of your parents share the same views on acquiring and saving things?
- Have you approached them about decluttering, and if so, what was their response?
- Are they on board with this plan for organizing and decluttering? [*Note*: I have a policy that I won't initiate a call to a potential client—they have to call my office and ask for help.]
- If they agree to getting help, do you think they would want you on site, or would having you there escalate the situation? Do you *want* to be there?

- To your knowledge, is your mother/father seeing a therapist for any type of mental health challenges? How about any medical challenges that might affect decision-making, mobility, etc.?
- Please be aware that you might be most helpful if you aren't part of the actual decluttering/organizing process. How would you feel if you just came at the end of the day to drive their donations to a destination of their choice instead of spending all day on site and possibly *not* being able to tolerate the rate of progress? (Sometimes it's painfully slow for bystanders.)
- Who will be paying for the services?

There is no easy way around this, but the initial conversation is non-negotiable in order for us to be able to provide the best services to our clients.

Therapist-Initiated Call

When therapists call, often they want to learn how organizers work in the home with their clients. They may see clients monthly, for years, and treat them for depression, ADHD, anger management, couples counseling, etc., but the therapist may have *no idea* of the squalor/conditions of their home. The client's shopping and acquiring habits are never discussed, go undiagnosed, and therefore are untreated. Unfortunately, I've seen this situation repeated more times than I can count. I know this happens because my clients tell me. It is worth noting that therapists listen to organizers, but they do not share any personal information that the client has shared with them; they honor confidentiality.

The Therapist-Organizer Conversation

When a therapist calls me, I may suggest that they ask for a photo of the client's living space so they can see it for themselves.

Therapists have different responses to this idea, but as I mentioned earlier, the proverbial picture is worth a thousand words.

There are two other common questions a therapist might ask me: How long will it take? How much does it cost? Neither have short answers.

How Long Will It Take?

It depends on the client's decision-making ability. Some want to give serious consideration and share stories about every scrap of paper, plastic grocery bag, and dead houseplant. Others want to have us do a pre-sort (where we group like objects together and "stage" the contents, then bring them in for what I call a "Round of One-Word Answers: Keep vs. Go." The latter, of course, means we accomplish a lot more, and I can give the client homework to do after we leave, saving them time and money.

How Much Does It Cost?

This depends on:
- How much stuff needs sorting and removing
- The number of people on the organizing team
- Who else needs to be called in on the job: exterminators, contractors, junk hauling teams, housecleaning crews, and so forth

Some clients *know* that it will take more time and more money if we keep the team small, but they oftentimes have trust issues and prefer to work at a slow, steady pace. They prefer the intimacy of one, two, or three organizers and can't bear the thought of a crew of strangers in their home—such as they may have seen on television.

We try to respect a client's wishes whenever possible in regard to the number of people involved. There are, unfortunately, always times when the law dictates that action has to be taken to remove a tenant from an apartment, or to remove children, elderly people, or pets from an unsafe home. Clients with hoarding disorders do not always make good neighbors in the sense that there are often rats, roaches, and smells from decaying food and neglected pets. In my experience, however, these clients are not dangerous in that they are not likely to harm themselves or another person.

In Perspective

As I mentioned earlier, should you ever contact Metropolitan Organizing, this chapter gives you a taste of what to expect. On the other hand, your experience with another professional organizer may be totally different. The important thing is to work with someone with whom you can connect and communicate. Do not be afraid to contact several professional organizers until you find the one who is right for you and your situation.

Wrapping Up and Moving On

From Hoarding to Hope: Understanding People Who Hoard and How to Help Them was never intended to be a complete compendium or reference book on hoarding disorder/tendencies. There is simply too much ever-changing information on the subject. However, I hope that the time you have spent reading *From Hoarding to Hope* has given you a different perspective on clutter, collecting, chronic disorganization, and hoarding disorder. I hope that you can now look beyond a hoard, really see the person buried beneath it, bring your compassionate understanding to the situation, and do what you can to help. If you find yourself coordinating an intervention, I hope you feel supported by knowing that there are resources available and how to choose the best members for your team.

Finally, if you are asked to be on a team in a hoarding situation (maybe it is your first experience), I hope that *From Hoarding to Hope* gives you the insights you need to begin. In Chapter 16, the next (and concluding) chapter, you will find additional resources. These include organizations and support groups, and suggested authors, videos, and Internet search terms to help get you started.

Chapter 16

Resources

Pre-Internet, a book like this would include an encyclopedia-type collection of available resources. However, there is so much information about hoarding disorder constantly being added, removed, and updated that *From Hoarding to Hope* would be out-of-date even before it went to press. Rather, I am being selective with my resources—not to limit your search for assistance, but because I am most familiar with these and can recommend them with confidence. Moreover, these resources also will be able to lead you to others.

Internet-search key terms to find an organizer near you:
professional organizers/hoarding/city

Organizations
- International OCD Foundation
- ICD (Institute for Challenging Disorganization)
- NAPO (National Association of Professional Organizers)
- POC (Professional Organizers in Canada)

- JALO (Japan Association of Life Organizers)
- APDO (Association of Professional Declutterers and Organisers)
- AAPO (Australasian Association of Professional Organisers)
- NPBO (Netherlands Professional Organizing Conference)

Clean out when no organizer needed

Service Master, ServiceMaster Clean, and SERVPRO are nationally recognized cleaning services whose employees have had special training. Check back in Chapter 14 for more information about when to call in specialized cleaning services.

Help in the community

Landlords and apartment managers: Check with your attorney for the best course of action.

Hoarding task forces

At this writing, there is no national task force on hoarding. See the International OCD Foundation for updated task force listings.

To seek help in your community
- *Start locally*: Town or City Clerk's Office, Board of Health, Council on Aging
- *Regionally*: If your local governmental agencies aren't able to offer help, try county or regional agencies.
- *State:* If you found no help at the local or regional level, try the state level. You also may be able to find colleges or universities that can give you direction.

Authors I recommend
- Belk, Russell
- Bratiotis, Christiana
- Frost, Randy
- Hartl, Tamara
- Steketee, Gail
- Tolin, David
- Tompkins, Michael

Groups to check out that may be helpful

Please note that I have no direct personal experience with these groups.

- Buried in Treasures Workshops
- Children of Hoarders
- Messies Anonymous
- Clutterers Anonymous

Questions to ask when hiring a professional organizer

1. What are your areas of expertise?
2. Are you certified? If so, by whom?
3. Are you insured?
4. Do you attend conferences or tele-classes and stay abreast of current trends and techniques?
5. Do you have local references?
6. Do you belong to any professional organizations?
7. How long have you been in business?
8. What hours do you work? What days of the week are you available?
9. Do you bring necessary supplies, or do I purchase them separately?

10. If you purchase supplies or materials, do you receive a discount?
11. Do you upcharge when buying items directly from vendors?
12. Do you have an hourly shopping rate?
13. How are supplies paid for: my credit card or yours?
14. Do you make arrangements to take away any donations, consignments, and trash? If so, do you charge a fee for this service?
15. Do you work alone, or do you have a team of employees or subcontractors if necessary?
16. Would you be willing to arrive in an unmarked vehicle?
17. Do you take photographs on my property?
18. Do you take before and after photographs?
19. With your camera or mine?
20. Do you use those photos in your marketing materials/website?
21. What is your fee, and how do you charge (per hour, per job, etc.)?
22. Do you charge a retainer fee?

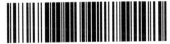

Made in the USA
Middletown, DE
18 September 2016